Your Health
It's a Question of Balance

If It Ain't Broke . . .

When it comes to quality of health and preventative medicine, the Western approach is off the mark. It denies the very existence of the parts of your body that are crucial to your vitality—your chi and your aura.

Time and time again I hear stories of people going to the doctor complaining that they "don't feel right." The doctor checks them the "modern" way, finds nothing wrong, and either sends them home with a "Tsk, tsk, it's all in your head," or with some medication to calm them so they don't notice that they are not feeling right. Most likely, these patients have recognized a blockage in their chi. If their chi is strengthened at this stage, it's likely that a more serious problem will be avoided and the day-to-day quality of their lives will be greatly improved, as will their energy levels.

When I was studying in China, a doctor told me, "In the West when you go to a doctor, they ask you about your family history. 'Did your parents suffer from any particular disease, for example?' Here in China, often the patients ask me, 'Is your family healthy? Are you in good health?' If I can't keep myself and my family in good health, why should a person put his life in my hands?"

Your good health is in your hands.

About the Author

Doctor Igor Cetojevic was born in Bugojno, Bosnia-Herzegovina in 1962. After completing his medical degree in Sarajevo in 1988, he studied Chinese Traditional Medicine at The European Center for Peace and Development in Belgrade, Yugoslavia.

Francesca Pinoni was born in San Francisco, California. In 1977, she earned a BA in Theater Arts from the University of California at Santa Cruz. Since 1994 she has been working closely with Igor to develop his work and communicate it to a broader audience.

To Write to the Author

If you wish to contact the author or would like more information about this book, please write to the author in care of Llewellyn Worldwide and we will forward your request. Both the author and publisher appreciate hearing from you and learning of your enjoyment of this book and how it has helped you. Llewellyn Worldwide cannot guarantee that every letter written to the author can be answered, but all will be forwarded. Please write to:

Dr. Igor Cetojevic and Francesca Pinoni
℅ Llewellyn Worldwide
P.O. Box 64383, Dept. K1-56718-121-X
St. Paul, MN 55164-0383, U.S.A.

Please enclose a self-addressed stamped envelope for reply, or $1.00 to cover costs. If outside U.S.A., enclose international postal reply coupon.

your Health

It's a Question of Balance

Dr. Igor Cetojevic
& Francesca Pinoni

2000
Llewellyn Publications
St. Paul, Minnesota 55164-0383, U.S.A.

FIRST EDITION
First Printing, 2000

Book design and editing by Karin Simoneau
Cover art and interior illustrations © 2000 by Jim Caputo
Cover design by Lisa Novak

Library of Congress Cataloging-in-Publication Data
Cetojevic, Igor, 1962-
    Your health: a question of balance / Igor Cetojevic &
    Francesca Pinoni.
      p. cm.
    Includes bibliographical references.
    ISBN 1-56718-121-X
    1. Alternative medicine. 2. Medicine, Chinese. 3. Vital
    force—Therapeutic use. I.
    Pinoni, Francesca, 1955-II. Title.

    R733.C48 2000
    615.5—dc21   00-056534

Llewellyn Worldwide does not participate in, endorse, or have any authority or responsibility concerning private business transactions between our authors and the public.

    All mail addressed to the author is forwarded but the publisher cannot, unless specifically instructed by the author, give out an address or phone number.

Llewellyn Publications
A Division of Llewellyn Worldwide, Ltd.
P.O. Box 64383, Dept. K1-56718-121-X
St. Paul, MN 55164-0383, U.S.A.
www.llewellyn.com

Printed in the United States of America

For our friends

Contents

Preface

I met Igor at my son's eighth birthday party, which was at my house. A mutual friend brought him along. After the cake and ice cream, Igor showed the children how a pendulum works. They were spellbound, as was I. When people were leaving, I went over to Igor and asked, "Can you teach me to do that?" "Yes, I can," he replied. So began the long road—full of potholes, roundabouts, and a lot of fun—that has led to our marriage and the writing of this book.

In the early days of our friendship (and my apprenticeship), I had to pay close attention to what Igor was telling me because his English, as he would say, "Is not so good." I carried around a little blue notebook that had "Notes from Dr. Igor" written on the front cover. So many interesting things would come up in the normal course of our conversations that I decided to take notes. This little blue notebook became the basis for this book.

I was raised in California and had always been health-conscious; I watched my diet and knew the importance of exercise. Although I knew that diet was important, I didn't really understand why, nor did I comprehend how the body worked. Everything that Igor told me had such a lovely simplicity and feeling of truth to it. I was hooked.

He explained, very simply, how energy works, how the different organs in the body work, and how easy it is to stay healthy if you know how—and are prepared to take responsibility for your own health. I followed his advice and I feel healthier now than I have ever felt in my life. I've watched other people follow his advice and make dramatic improvements in their health and happiness.

It is with this insight and passion that we would like to share this information with you.

FRANCESCA PINONI

△△△△△△△△△△△

Introduction

I would like to explain my strategy of healing. I am qualified as a Medical Doctor, General Practitioner. When I completed my studies and started to practice medicine, I found that something was missing. Although I had been trained well and had good knowledge of Western medicine, I felt that it did not provide sufficient information to effectively heal my patients. It wasn't enough to prescribe medicine to patients and send them home to wait for the outcome—a practice that seemed to be the essence of Western medicine. Sometimes this method worked and sometimes it didn't, and when it didn't then another medicine would be tried. It seemed like a lot of trial and error. The patients would be lucky if the side effects of the "cure" were less uncomfortable than their original condition. What effect does this have on the physical and mental health of the patient?

Thank goodness I had the opportunity to learn about Chinese traditional medicine and acupuncture, which I studied for two years in Belgrade, Yugoslavia; I then took advanced courses in Beijing, China. From those studies, I learned how to look at patients' problems from a totally different perspective.

I learned about a "whole-system" philosophy that takes into account the entire person, rather than a system that views the body as a machine and attempts to fix its individual parts. Chinese medicine focuses on identifying and treating the *root cause* of a problem rather than merely alleviating the symptoms. This process sometimes takes a little longer but, in the long run, proves to be a much more efficient method of treatment. Once the root cause has been eliminated, a person will remain healthy. When only the symptom is treated, the problem will resurface either as the same condition or a different one based on the same root cause.

One education gave me one body of information; the other education gave me another; but even with all this information, I knew something was missing. As a child, I would drive my parents crazy by always asking "Why?" and "What?" over and over again. I guess it is this insatiable curiosity that prompts me to always be on the lookout for more information, more knowledge, and more pieces of the puzzle that will eventually add up to maximum health.

One day while I was studying in Beijing, China, I was sitting at the lunch table with a Chinese doctor. We talked about the difference between Chinese and Western medicine. He pointed to a teapot and said, "Look at the teapot . . . tell me about it." I answered, "It's white; it has a spout to pour the tea." "Anything else?" he asked me. "No." "What about the pink flower?" He turned the teapot around and I saw that there was a flower painted on that side. "If we look at things from different ways, we can observe different things. We could argue for hours about whether the teapot was solid white or if it had a flower on it. We are both right, from our individual perspectives. But look how much more we know when we share our observations and our points of view."

After studying both Western and Eastern healing systems, I encountered a very special doctor while attending a seminar in Belgrade. His name was Dr. Nikola Videv and he showed me, for the first time in my life, the etheric body. We covered many topics in Dr. Videv's class: acupuncture meridians, energy, chi, the Tao, aura, the etheric body—lots of interesting material. During one of the classes, he discussed vibrational medicine and dowsing. That was the first time I had ever heard about these things. I'd seen people fooling around with pendulums but I always thought it was silly. This time, however, I had a strong feeling that this information was something that would play an important role in my life.

I was impressed that a respected doctor, whose specialty was psychiatry, would stand up in front of a group of advanced students, all qualified doctors, many of them over fifty years old, and talk to us about such things as dowsing and vibrational medicine. It's often difficult for medical doctors to open doors and windows to let in fresh air.

Dr. Videv stood in front of the class and said, "Dear friends, I will show you something that would be very interesting for you to practice." He showed us two ordinary metal rods, about eighteen inches long, bent at right angles like an L. With his elbows near the sides of his body, he held the rods so that they were parallel to the floor. Then he walked across the classroom and something happened: At certain spots in the room the ends of the rods came together. As he kept walking they separated again. Why was that happening? Was the doctor moving the rods? If so, why? What's going on? Again . . . why and what?!

Then he took out a chain with a small metal cone attached: a pendulum. He put one hand on his heart and held the chain of the pendulum between the thumb and index finger of his other hand. Again he walked around the room. In some places the pendulum spun around in a circle. In other places it stopped moving. Why?

Dr. Videv explained that he was using the L-rods and pendulum as tools to make the unseen vibrations in the environment visible. He went on to talk about the effect that these vibrations have on our health and the health of our patients. This information touched me deeply and I would now like to share it with you. Neither Western nor Eastern medicine takes into consideration the influence of vibrations around us when looking into a patient's condition. These disturbing vibrations are caused by natural conditions in the earth or by manmade electrical equipment.

He shared how he observed this influence in the course of his work in a psychiatric hospital. "I was working in a hospital and had the idea to check the vibrations in the location of my patients' beds. One bed was in a spot that had a particularly harmful vibrational influence. I observed that patients who were in that particular bed suffered more acute symptoms than their neighbors in the ward who had similar complaints and were on similar medication. When these patients were moved to another bed, however, their condition immediately improved." Dr. Videv explained that people with psychiatric problems are more sensitive to vibrations around them; their threshold of sensitivity is higher than average. For example, when a light is switched on near them, they react more strongly than others would. Being in a place of strong negative vibration is like a slap to them.

Dr. Videv told us, "It is difficult to explain this briefly, but if some of you practice yoga or meditation, you may find it easier to use these tools." His words touched me again because I was interested in both yoga and meditation. I was sitting in the front row and eagerly volunteered to try the tools that he had shown us. He explained that for them to work we must keep our minds out of the picture and not expect anything to happen. I took the rods and walked across the room. I felt them moving in my hands! I knew that I had not consciously moved them and felt exhilarated because I was actually doing it. Dr. Videv looked me in the eye and said, "I think you are a good receiver. It is necessary for you to start slowly and check many places. You need years to be sure you know what you are doing." Now, after many years of checking space and people, I am sure of what I am doing! And I would like to offer my knowledge to you.

What did I do with the information I acquired from Dr. Videv? I applied his methods to my own system of treating patients by using acupuncture and herbs. As a result, their energy levels increased. Sometimes patients would respond well to treatment, but the next day their energy would drop and they would feel bad again. I compare the body to a rechargeable battery: During the treatment the battery fills up with energy; however, something causes the battery to leak energy. I knew my patients were following my instructions regarding proper food and medicinal herbs, so what was the problem? Why weren't the patients getting better? Again, why and what? I remembered Dr. Videv's lecture and decided to check the places where my patients spent a lot of time—the places where they slept and worked. Invariably, the patients who were not retaining the energy that was built up during their treatments were spending considerable time in places with strong negative vibrational influences. When they moved their beds or desks to a better position, their condition improved dramatically. They no longer lost the energy they acquired and they were able to add more energy with each additional treatment.

My mother is a teacher. Once I went to visit her at school. During recess I checked her classroom and found one particularly bad spot. Without letting on why I wanted to know, I asked, "Mom, who sits here?" "Oh," she said, "One very naughty boy. He can never sit still. He's always on the edge of his chair." Obviously, he was trying to get away from that spot which emitted disturbing vibrations. I asked her to move his desk to another spot, which she did and, as if by magic, his behavior changed. He was less restless and his concentration improved. Children have strong instincts, like animals. They are open. They like something or they don't. They do not like places with disturbing vibrations and will do whatever they can to get away from them.

On another occasion I was treating a woman at her home in Belgrade. It was difficult for her to relax during her treatment because her twin infant daughters would not stop crying. When I asked her why they cried so much, she said that she did not know; she had taken them to several doctors and was told that there was nothing wrong with them. They were a happy and financially stable family. There was no apparent reason for the babies to cry so much. I asked her to show me where they slept. When I checked the room, I found that both of their cribs were in very bad spots. I noticed that one of the cribs had an unusually high side and asked their mother about it. She said, "My baby kept rolling off the bed. We had to make the side higher to keep her in. The other baby sleeps huddled up in the corner of her crib." I advised the mother to move the cribs to the other side of the room, out of the areas that had strong vibrations. She agreed and the two of us moved the cribs. The next week I went to her home to treat her. She looked much better and was more relaxed. I had hardly walked through the door when she told me, "My neighbor came by yesterday and asked me, 'Where are your babies?' They have been so quiet since we moved their beds that the neighbors thought they weren't here anymore!"

Since then, I have observed time and time again that by locating the places of negative vibrational influence and repositioning the furniture so that one does not spend a lot of time in there, many chronic symptoms disappear.

I also use the pendulum to check the energy of my patients. The pendulum is my "x-ray." It shows me where the patient's weaknesses are and how they are responding to treatment. When I check a patient, I use a lot of synonyms for what I am measuring: temperature, bioenergy, etheric body, and aura. This is nothing new. Some people can see the human aura. I can feel it.

It is important to me that my patients know I am a medical doctor and have gained a lot of knowledge from both Western and Eastern medical traditions. When a patient comes to see me, I tell him or her, "You are not my patient, you are my friend. I ask you to take *responsibility* for your body, mind, and spirit. Using all my knowledge, I will do my best to help you. However, in the end, it is your body and your responsibility to take care of it. There is a big problem today with people not taking responsibility for themselves. Some people expect their physicians to "fix" them when they become ill. They seem to have the attitude that they can eat all the junk food they see advertised on television, smoke, and lead an inactive life, and when they get sick the insurance company will cover the cost of making them better. If they don't get better, they sometimes blame the doctors because, after all, they are being paid to cure them. Well, it doesn't work that way.

I liken my view of healing to this sign:

If I use all my knowledge and do my best work, the maximum I can contribute is one-third of the whole picture.

If my patients follow my recommendations and take responsibility for their own healing process, then add another third.

Two-thirds is more than halfway there. Our combined human effort in coming this far invites help from a higher power. The last third is in the hands of God.

I would like to teach people how to take responsibility for their third. In this book, I will explain, very simply, what it takes to create your own health. I'll show you the pieces of the puzzle that, when gathered together, can create total health. It's really very simple—when you know how. That's what this book is about.

Let's go!

1

▲▲▲▲▲▲▲▲▲▲▲

In the Beginning

You've seen this sign: a black and white circle with a design that resembles two fish swimming head to tail. Do you know what it means?

For our purpose, let's call this the Yin/Yang Sign. It is the basis of understanding *dynamic balance*, and balance is the key to health. Pretty simple so far.

All things in this world can be viewed as either Yin or Yang, two opposite things that cannot exist without each other. The shape of the sign signifies both unity and motion. Nothing is static. What is Yin is now moving toward becoming Yang, and what is Yang is moving toward becoming Yin. You say, "This isn't so simple . . . "

Here's an example: Think of a year starting from the middle of winter. This is as Yin as it gets. It's cold, it's dark, the days are short, and the nights are long. As the months pass, soon it is springtime. At the time of the spring equinox, the lengths of the day and the night are the same. The temperatures are mild, neither hot nor cold. There is a moment of perfect equilibrium, and then what happens? There is a shift to the Yang side. The days become hotter and longer until midsummer. What happens then? Does it get hotter and hotter? No, the balance starts to shift again as fall follows summer with another moment of equilibrium until Yin begins to predominate again. And so it goes, over and over again, year in and year out.

So, what? First, you can see that the ratio of Yin to Yang changes as the earth moves through her seasonal changes, and this cycle repeats itself indefinitely. Second, you have learned some of the properties of Yin (cold, dark) and Yang (hot, light). Third, a state of balance is not static; everything moves and changes and still preserves its balance. Fourth, and a little more subtly, you may have realized that the varying amount of Yin and Yang through the course of the year might very well have an effect on our health.

I'll be using this seesaw a lot. It clearly illustrates the idea of dynamic balance.

Yin and Yang are foreign words. Try to think of Yin as being a magnetic or contracting force (like gravity, something that pulls something into itself), and Yang as being a dynamic or expanding force (like centrifugal force, which is what you see in a clothes dryer; it is the force that pushes things away from itself).

Take a moment to observe yourself. How are you sitting right now? You can learn a lot from your body.

This is a Yang position.

This is a Yin position.

How come and what does it mean? I'll explain.

Here are some attributes of Yin and Yang:

Yin	Yang
Feminine	Masculine
Cold	Hot
Wet	Dry
Closing	Opening
Contraction	Expansion
Stillness	Movement
Dark	Light
Magnetic	Dynamic
Sweet	Salty

Sweet? Salty? What's this? Well, I'm sneaking in something important here.

Let's take a look at food. We need food to live. We need food to get the vitamins, minerals, proteins, carbohydrates, and fats that we use to energize and build our bodies. We need the right food to be healthy. You may be asking, "Why is he giving us information that is just common sense?" I know . . . you know these things already. But *what is the right food?*

There is no right food. Wait! Don't stone me yet! There is "right food," but it is not the same right food for everybody, at all times. Remember what I said at the start of this chapter: Balance is the key.

More than likely, you have been taught from an early age that maintaining a balanced diet and eating nutritious food is good for you. You learned the basic information about a balanced diet as a child when you were in elementary school and the rules were emphasized during adolescence when you were in high school. You were probably taught by your parents and teachers and other influential people in your life the importance of nutrition. Well . . . eating balanced meals is a good start. Just what is a balanced meal? A balanced meal is considered to consist of foods from the different food groups: starches, meat, fruit and vegetables, and so forth. But that's not enough in itself. This simplified formula does not take into consideration other important factors like the type of work you do, the climate in which you live, or the weather, for example.

I can hear you now: "You said this would be *simple,* but if I have to think about all these things, it won't be simple at all." Before you give up, just slow down and keep reading.

Let's go back to our illustration of the seesaw:

Here is the seesaw showing Yin and Yang as the extreme points. Our aim is to keep our balance.

When it is time to eat, there are certain things to consider with a view toward this seesaw. These things are:

- The relative position of the weather

- The relative position of the type of work that you are doing

- The relative position of the food on the seesaw

That's not so much, now, is it?

Let's start with the weather since you all know when it's cold outside.

Here's the seesaw. Hot is on the Yang side; cold is on the Yin side:

This is a very hot summer day in Mexico.

This is a snowy winter day in Alaska.

And this is a lovely day for a picnic.

Next, let's look at the work we do. Some of us have jobs that require hard physical labor, such as constructing buildings, farming, or herding cows; but most of us have pretty sedentary jobs these days.

Here's a cowboy. Being a cowboy requires lots of activity. Physical work depleted his Yang energy and he needs more Yang food to make the seesaw balance.

Here's an accountant. Being an accountant requires lots of brainwork. Mental work depleted his Yin energy and he needs more Yin food to balance the seesaw.

Do you find it easy to go outside and have a strenuous workout on a very hot day? No way. Why? Because there is too much Yang in that equation. You literally burn up. Is it a coincidence that people who live in hot countries often take a siesta in the afternoon? I don't think so.

Now we come to food. This one is a little less obvious for those of us who grew up in the Western world. No one ever told us that some foods are Yin and others are Yang . . . stay with me. You learned to count calories, which is a whole lot easier.

To put it simply, if a food is salty it is Yang. If it is sweet it is Yin. Here's a list starting with foods that are closest to the center of the seesaw. I'll save the irregular ones for last. These must be memorized, just like French verbs (but tastier).

Yin	Yang
Grains	Milk
Cereal	Mushrooms
Seeds (sesame, sunflower)	Beans
Yogurt	Soy Products
Oil (from seeds)	Cheese
Vegetables	Chicken
Garlic	Olive Oil
Fruit	Fish
Tropical Fruit	Nuts
Fruit Juice	Beef
Sweets	Pork
Vinegar	Eggs
Alcohol	Salt
White Sugar	Onions*
Almonds*	Carrots*
	Beets*

*Exception to the rules

Generally speaking, salt is extreme Yang, proteins (such as red meat) are strong Yang, and fats are moderate Yang. Carbohydrates (such as grains and cereals) are moderate Yin, vitamins and minerals are Yin, sweets are strong Yin, and white sugar is Yin to the max.

With a little practice, you can use a pendulum to test whether food is Yin or Yang. If you don't happen to have a pendulum lying around the house, a key or a ring tied on a piece of string that is about five inches long works just fine. Practice first with unmarked salt and sugar.

Sit comfortably at your dining table. Have two identical bowls ready, one with a tablespoon of sugar in it and another with a tablespoon of salt. Put your elbow on the table and hold the chain of the pendulum between your thumb and index finger. Hold it over the bowl containing the sugar and observe the movement of the pendulum. Relax your shoulders, elbows, and wrists, and be patient. Keep breathing. Next, hold the pendulum over the salt. After a while, you should observe a different movement. Make a note of the direction the pendulum moves for sugar (Yin) and salt (Yang). The movements are not the same for everyone, so you'll need to do this test first.

Just for fun, have someone change the position of the bowls so you don't know which one is which. Test the two bowls again and then check and see if you identified them correctly. If not, try again. And don't forget to breathe. This doesn't work if you hold your breath. Remember to be patient, as this can take some practice.

Once you and your pendulum can identify the sugar and salt, then you are ready to check other foods to see if they produce Yin or Yang energy.

Not all foods are created equal. Here is our friendly seesaw showing the relative positions of different Yin and Yang foods. As you get proficient with the pendulum, it will make bigger movements for foods that are close to the extremes.

Rice and grains are just about in the center. These are balanced foods and combine well with other foods. Spring water is as good as it gets. Water helps balance the foods you eat. Have you noticed that when you eat very salty food or very sweet food you feel very thirsty? Now you know why. Your body as asking for *balance*.

The idea is to create a meal that will perfectly balance the seesaw. You may think that you can do that by eating only brown rice (remember the macrobiotic diet?), but it doesn't quite work that way.

Some of you might be thinking, "Oh, good. If I drink whiskey with my spareribs I'll have a perfect balance." Not quite. If you try to make a balance from *extreme* Yin and Yang, it doesn't work.

Regarding the rice-only diet, it doesn't work unless you live in a perfect climate all year 'round, you do just enough mental and physical work, and you don't have any stress or emotional ups and downs. Why? Let's see. It's time to put everything together on that handy little seesaw.

The starting point.

It's summer. It's a hot day.

Add a bowl of chili and we hit bottom.

Way too Yang. So what do you do?

You go to sleep, which is an extreme Yin activity.

If you wanted to spend the rest of the day having fun at the beach instead of fast asleep in your bed, a more balanced meal would be a fresh salad and iced tea.

Bon appetit!

Now, close your eyes if you will and try to imagine a vegetarian Eskimo. Too Yin. Or how about a South Sea Islander chomping on spareribs and stew. It just does not compute.

Pretty simple, isn't it?

2

△△△△△△△△△△△

Ups and Downs

I started this book with an example of the yearly cycle. Now I will show you how the different cycles of the year, even of each day, provide clues that will help you to keep yourself in top shape. First, here's a little lesson.

Chinese Medicine 1A

All our organs are either Yin or Yang. How can you tell which is which? It's pretty easy. The Yin organs are generally compact and more solid, and the Yang organs are hollow and let things flow through them.

Every organ has a buddy. They make a cooperative couple; one Yin organ with one Yang organ. Each pair of organs is associated with an opening in your face. So, be aware that you are showing your state of health to anyone who knows where to look. Pretty soon you will know where to look, too.

Each pair of organs is also associated with an emotion. Emotion! What do emotions have to do with the physical body? Plenty, as we will see later.

Each season of the year is associated with one pair of organs.

As you can see, each pair of organs has its own season. What does this mean? This means that if you have a predisposition for a weakness in an organ, the problem will most likely occur during its own season. Organs work harder in their own season. More people suffer from heart attacks in the summer than at any other time of the year. Asthma, a condition of the lungs, is more prevalent in the autumn. When the seasons change, pay attention to your stomach and spleen.

When you have this knowledge, you can save yourself a lot of hassle and expense by strengthening your body *before* the beginning of each new season. Don't forget that *prevention is the highest medicine.* You can prevent the worsening of a chronic condition and stop problems that develop because of weak organs by beginning treatment a month *before* the season associated with that organ.

For example, if you suffer from respiratory problems (such as asthma, bronchitis, pneumonia, or emphysema), they will probably flare up in autumn. Therefore, head them off at the pass by strengthening your lungs at the end of summer before autumn, lung season, begins. If you suffer from kidney ailments, sciatica, or lumbago, begin treatment in autumn (before the cold days begin) to prevent a flare-up in winter.

What type of treatment would be appropriate? A healthy diet is the first thing to consider. (That's why chapter 1 was all about food.) There are also various herbs that are great in supporting the various organs. There is a lot of material out there about the healing power of herbs. Before you go forward and begin using herbs as a treatment, do some research and read as much information as you can about herbs, their uses, and the benefits they have to offer.

Let's get back to Yin and Yang. Remember our friends from chapter 1?

Here is a Yin position.

Here is a Yang position.

Now, take a look at yourself. If you generally sit with your arms and legs crossed, if you often feel cold, if you are very thin, if you don't talk too much, or if you don't have to run to the bathroom very often, then your body is more Yin and you are more likely to develop a Yin (cold) ailment in moments of weakness.

All stiffness in the body is Yin. For example, colds, chilly fingers and toes, muscle and joint stiffness, and depression are all signs of too much Yin in your body.

If you are very active, speak loudly, perspire a lot, often feel hot, sit with your arms and legs apart, are quick to react, and tend to be emotional, then your body has more Yang and you will be more likely to develop a Yang (hot) ailment.

All excess heat in the body is Yang. For example, fever, excess perspiration, thirst, nervousness, and constipation are signs that there's too much Yang in your body.

Of course, like most things, this isn't black and white. These examples are extreme cases and people change according to circumstances. However, take it as a guideline and follow me.

Look out the window. What kind of a day is it out there? When the weather is humid, the body becomes "sticky." All the water in the body is sticky, not liquid; it is more like oil. Traveling to a humid climate and not adjusting your food accordingly results in lethargy and heaviness. The body needs some stimulation to achieve better balance.

When the weather is hot and humid, drink tea that is Yin and eat fresh fruit and salads to ease the flow of liquid in your body. Heavy foods like meat and rich foods like dairy products create a "stickiness" in your body. It is important that you use small amounts of salt and sugar. These are two extreme substances and will create an "internal steam bath" by collecting water, which the body cannot control. The water will be retained in the body, resulting in swollen legs and a bloated, heavy feeling. Eat light foods and drink lots of spring water.

If the day is cold and rainy, enjoy a hearty stew or bake a batch of delicious gingersnaps. You'll find the recipe at the end of the book.

Coffee and Tea

I'm not going to tell you that you should never drink coffee. I can hear the sighs of relief. I do want you to be aware of *when* you drink it and what happens to you when you do.

Coffee is Yin but it has a Yang manifestation in your body. How's that for a twist? A cup of coffee stimulates your body by creating little spasms in your small blood vessels that raise your blood pressure and wake you up.

Hot English tea (black tea) works the same way. It's good to drink it in places that have a cold, damp climate, such as England. Well . . . fancy that.

Green tea (Chinese tea) is Yin. It calms the body and is good to drink in hot, humid climates, such as southern China.

Tannin in tea and caffeine in coffee are *drugs.* All drugs, if overused, can cause the body to shake. Sometimes the body needs a little stimulation, but remember that these substances are strong; use them consciously.

Now is a good time to mention "demon alcohol." If you drink alcohol, which is Yin, in moderation, it can be useful to stimulate Yin organs such as the pancreas and liver to produce digestive juices, which help to digest food. If you slip from moderate use to excessive use, alcohol will damage those organs.

Any chronic excess of either Yin or Yang will damage your system.

Food controls the balance, which is precisely why it is so important. You can choose the food you eat much more easily than you can control the weather.

Now let's talk about another cycle: day and night. Guess what time is the most Yang?

That's right. Noon is the most Yang time of day. The sun is at its strongest. After noon, the sun has passed its highest point and the day progresses toward night. Midnight is the most Yin time, when all the world is quiet and dark.

It's useful to know that the Chinese associate different times of day with the different organs of the body;

at two-hour intervals, different organs are at their peak energy level.

Here is a chart that shows which organs are associated with the hours of the day. The day is divided into twelve two-hour parts. Each part has one organ. Knowing which is which is very helpful in finding out the root cause of a problem. I'll explain more about how this works later. For now, take a look at the chart.

Time	Organ	Association
5 A.M. to 7 A.M	Large Intestine	If you need to use the restroom now, it's a sign of good health
7 A.M. to 9 A.M.	Stomach	Eat breakfast
9 A.M. to 11 A.M.	Spleen	Digest your breakfast
11 A.M. to 1 P.M.	Heart	Coffee time
1 P.M. to 3 P.M.	Small Intestine	Lunch time
3 P.M. to 5 P.M.	Urine Bladder	Liquid out
5 P.M. to 7 P.M.	Kidney	Teatime (liquid in)
7 P.M. to 9 P.M.	Pericardium	Light meal
9 P.M. to 11 P.M.	Triple Heater	Time to relax
11 P.M. to 1 A.M.	Gall Bladder	Nighty-night
1 A.M. to 3 A.M.	Liver	Your body is rebuilding now
3 A.M. to 5 A.M.	Lungs	Sweet dreams

On the following page is an illustration containing information similar to that which is in the chart, but the illustration may give you a clearer understanding of the relationship between the time of day and specific organ functions. You will also see that certain times of the day are more Yin and certain times of the day are more Yang.

Think for a moment about some of these questions: Is there a certain time of the day when your energy seems lower? At what time do you seem to have the most energy? Do you regularly wake up at a particular time during the night? Are you more apt to use the restroom in the morning? In the evening? After evaluating some of these things, refer to the chart and see which organ correlates with that time. If, for instance, you are waking up at a certain time every night, make note of the time, find it on the chart, and you will see the organ that is associated with that time. More than likely you have a little weakness in that organ. Great. Now that you know about it, you can support that organ so it doesn't have to get really sick before you *do something* for it.

"What do I do?" you ask.

Ups and Downs

First of all, *observe* yourself. Get used to paying attention to what is going on in your body at different times of the day. For example, look at 5 A.M. to 7 A.M. on the chart. That is the time of the large intestine. In other words, it's more or less the correct time to go to the bathroom and "empty the recycling bin." If you are in a state of good health, then you are probably, naturally and easily, eliminating your personal waste products daily around this time.

If you suffer from constipation, it is a sign that your intestines are dry. Because dryness is a Yang condition, you need more Yin food like fresh fruits and vegetables because they will create moisture in your system. Are you beginning to see how this works?

If you have the opposite condition and suffer from diarrhea, it is a sign that you have an excess of dampness, an extreme Yin condition, in your intestines. Wet, wet, wet. You need to gradually increase the Yang energy by drinking a cup of strong black tea (without sugar) and boiling up a hot stew of carrots and rice.

If you need a clothespin to put on your nose or you have to leave the bathroom window wide open, maybe you should give a thought to your digestion: Strong odor comes from undigested foods, especially animal proteins. Be aware that the process of digestion starts in your mouth. Eat slowly and chew your food well so you get a head start on digestion. There's more about the digestive process in the next chapter.

5 A.M. **to** 7 A.M. is Large Intestine Time. As mentioned before, this is the appropriate time to use the restroom. If you are a healthy individual, you are more than likely eliminating waste products around this time naturally.

7 A.M. **to** 9 A.M. is Stomach Time. This is the time to have a nourishing breakfast. Don't skip this meal; it provides your fuel for the day. The food you eat in the morning has the best chance of being completely digested. Maybe the Australians are on the right track—they eat steak and eggs for breakfast.

9 A.M. **to** 11 A.M. is Spleen Time. One of the spleen's functions is to support the stomach and finish off the digestive process that is started. I'll tell you more about the spleen in the next chapter.

11 A.M. **to** 1 P.M. is Heart Time. Bitter taste feeds the heart, so if you want a cup of coffee, this is a good time to have it. As a matter of fact, in England, work stops for "Elevenses," which is what they call their midmorning coffee break.

1 P.M. **to** 3 P.M. is Small Intestine Time. In other words, a good time to eat lunch.

3 P.M. **to** 5 P.M. is Urine Bladder Time. Your bladder is most active at this time. It is getting pretty full and it's time to visit the bathroom and get rid of the liquid waste.

5 P.M. **to** 7 P.M. is Kidney Time. A cup of herbal tea increases the fluid in your body and will help to flush out your kidneys. It's also a good time for a catnap.

7 P.M. **to** 9 P.M. is Pericardium Time. The pericardium is the sack that surrounds and protects the heart. I'll tell you more about your pericardium in the next chapter. For now, it's enough to know that this is the time to unwind, to calm down after your busy day, and a good time to cuddle your partner.

9 P.M. **to** 11 P.M. is Triple Heater Time. It's best not to eat too much during this time—you don't want to burn your triple heater. The triple heater is similar to what Western medicine calls "the autonomic nervous system." It controls and balances all the other organs, supporting them with energy. This is the time when the body's automatic systems begin to work harder, processing the intake of the day and rebalancing your body by night.

11 P.M. **to** 1 A.M. is Gall Bladder Time. Have you ever had the experience of not being able to sleep after eating a particularly heavy dinner? This is your gall bladder running on overdrive; the hum of its motor keeps you awake.

1 A.M. to 3 A.M. is Liver Time. Your liver, the main factory in your body, is active at this time. If you often have disturbing dreams and wake up at this time, your liver probably needs some support.

3 A.M. to 5 A.M. is Lung Time. This is the time of deep, deep sleep. While you slumber, your lungs are working hard. Oxygen is the connection between the inside of your body and the outside environment. Most of the nutrients from the food you eat need oxygen to convert them into energy that your body can use. If you wake up at this time wheezing or have trouble breathing, there's probably a weakness of energy in your lungs.

This brings us back to 5 A.M. to 7 A.M.—Large Intestine Time. Good morning!

It's best not to eat too much in the evening. This is a time when the body's automatic systems begin to work harder, processing the intake of the day and rebalancing your body throughout night. Notice the time that you wake up during the night, especially if it's every night. It may indicate a weakness in the organ that relates to the time that your sleep is disturbed. For example, if you always wake up around 3 A.M., your liver probably needs some support.

If you have any sort of infection (common symptoms of infections are a temperature, sore throat, runny nose, diarrhea, or vaginal discharge), don't feed it sugar. Bacteria and viruses that cause infections thrive on sugar and sweets. If you want them to go away, starve them by taking away their favorite food.

Garlic is *great*. Use garlic during the cold and flu season to prevent infections. It is a natural antibiotic. Garlic also helps to lower high blood pressure by dissolving accumulated fat and cholesterol. In addition, it stimulates digestion. Add one or two cloves of fresh garlic near the end of cooking. Do not overcook garlic, as this will destroy some of its healthful properties.

Some helpful herbs and spices that you may already have in your kitchen:

Chamomile: A cup of chamomile tea is very good for digestive problems, insomnia, and menstrual cramps. It stabilizes and calms the energy of the stomach and intestines. If your tummy is upset in the morning (stomach hours), then drink chamomile tea. It's very good for soothing the discomfort of morning sickness. You can also use chamomile tea for eye irritations. Put some warm (not hot) tea on a piece of cotton and bathe your eyelids.

Mint: Mint tea relaxes and cools the body. It promotes circulation of bile in the liver and gall bladder and relieves discomfort in the upper right-hand side of the abdomen, where it disperses accumulated energy and can help relieve a migraine headache if the root of the headache is in the liver and gall bladder (more on this subject later). If you feel uncomfortable late at night and in the early hours of the morning, then try drinking a cup of mint tea. It works great to ease a hangover. Even better, if you can remember to drink a cup between alcoholic beverages, then you can avoid a hangover altogether. (How do I know this? I have to admit it's through personal experience.)

Cinnamon: This spice is *numero uno* (the best) for promoting circulation in the heart. It warms the entire body, creating a kind of internal central heating system. You can use cinnamon sticks to brew a pot of tea. Add powdered cinnamon to coffee, cocoa, or even food.

Licorice: Drinking licorice tea cleanses and detoxifies the body. It stimulates both the spleen and stomach and supports the digestive system. It is also very good for children who have a lack of appetite. By regularly drinking licorice tea, toxins are eliminated before they can cause damage to the body. Licorice is a great preventative and curative medicine—and it tastes good, too.

Ginger: This spice warms the body and helps digestion. It also warms the stomach, spleen, and intestines. If you have a weakness in your digestive system, drink a cup of ginger tea between 7 A.M. and 11 A.M., the times of your stomach and spleen.

Speaking of the spleen . . . who knows what the spleen
does? Or what a gall bladder does besides make stones
that shouldn't be there? For a simple introduction to
the inner you—read on.

3

△△△△△△△△△△△

Upon Closer Look

now I will give you a little bit of information about what is going on inside of you. It's time to meet the in-laws; those strange and unfamiliar beings that are a part of the family but not very familiar.

One cell from a woman and one cell from a man meet. They swim together in a beautiful dance of life. What do they do?

Two cells join together to create a new motion of life.

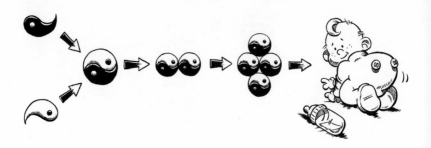

Through motion, they expand their life force and divide and multiply: the two become four, the four become sixteen, the sixteen become 256, and so on and so on. After about three months, there is a teeny, tiny little one swimming around in its mother's womb; a little fish with its mother's eyes and its father's nose.

This motion is called *Organogenisis* or, for those who don't speak Greek, "the Birth of the Organs." By three months, all of the major organs have formed. They continue to grow and develop, each as a vital part of the whole, holy human. Let's take a look at some parts of the human body and the role these parts play.

Kidneys

Your kidneys are the "boss." They hold the genetic blue-prints that have the instructions on how everything else works and are the main battery of the body—the power source that keep things going. One of the boss's duties is to filter your blood. Your kidneys remove toxins from your blood and allow what remains to continue traveling around your body providing fuel for your cells. The toxins are eliminated in the form of urine, which is stored in your urine bladder until it's time to go . . . to the bathroom. Your kidneys control the function of your ears, bones, joints, and reproductive organs.

Lungs

Your lungs are the processing plant for oxygen, one of your body's two main fuels. Our first and last connection with the outside world is through a *breath*. Oxygen in the air is processed by the lungs and sent to all your cells via your blood as it circulates through your body, dropping off oxygen and collecting carbon dioxide. It returns to the lungs where the carbon dioxide is removed and leaves your body when you exhale. *Aaahhh!* Your lungs control the quality of your skin.

Heart

Your heart pumps blood all throughout your body. Your blood carries oxygen in and carbon dioxide out and also regulates your body's temperature. It transports nutrients from the food you eat into your cells and carries waste products away. Oxygen and nutrients are the two fuels that keep your body running.

The Chinese say, "Your spirit dwells in your heart." What does that mean? It means that the energy of your heart inspires your deepest thoughts and dreams. Love is the energy of your heart; your spirit. The energy of your heart is expressed verbally by what you say and how you say it. Free and relaxed communication makes you lighthearted and happy.

Pericardium

Your pericardium (what's that?) is a type of sack around your heart. I think of it as a nest that cuddles and protects your heart, helping it do its job of circulating your blood.

Stomach

Your stomach breaks down proteins and prepares other food so it can be absorbed and enter your blood in a form that the body can use. The process of digestion starts in your mouth. When you chew your food well, saliva is produced. The action of saliva on the food starts the digestive process. When lunch reaches your stomach the fluids there break down the proteins. The proteins, which are now broken up into little pieces, and the rest of the food, which isn't (especially if you ate quickly and didn't chew it well), go into the small intestine.

Small Intestine

Your small intestine is the main place where food is absorbed. Close your eyes and picture a twenty-foot-long hose coiled up in your belly. Imagine the tube lined with fur. Your blood flows into the tiny strands and picks up the nutrients that have been absorbed by the small intestine. Spy cells are on the lookout for fat. When they identify fat, they get on their cell phones and call your gall bladder.

Gall Bladder

Your gall bladder sends a shot of bile into the small intestine. Bile is a digestive juice that breaks down fat so that it can be absorbed by the small intestine. (Imagine a turkey baster squirting out a shot of bile.) The proteins that were broken down in the stomach continue to be digested and are absorbed into the small intestine; from there they flow into your bloodstream.

Liver

All the nutrient-rich blood must pass through your liver, the body's main factory. This is where all the magic happens. Your digestive system breaks down the food you eat into its basic components. In your liver, all these building blocks are reassembled into a kind of nuclear fuel. All the various types of fuel that the different parts of your body require are constructed in your liver—the master chef that turns the raw ingredients into your personal favorite dish. The whole smorgasbord is served up through your bloodstream, and each part of your body takes what it needs to energize and build it.

Your liver cleans your blood and recycles it. In addition to this, it stores extra blood that is not currently needed for circulation, acting rather like a Fort Knox for the body, providing essential reserves in case of massive blood loss through injury. Your liver produces the bile that is stored in the gall bladder; this bile is used to break down fat. And look! The state that your liver is in also has an effect on your eyes and your vision. Evaluating these two things is a good way to measure the condition of this organ.

Yet another way to assess the quality of your liver is to look at your nails. If they are strong and healthy, so is your liver.

Spleen

Your spleen is a storehouse for blood that may be needed in an emergency. In case of infection, your spleen sends troops of white blood cells to the rescue. Your spleen is also the "old folks home" for blood. After traveling around your body for three or four months, red blood cells go to your spleen to relax and take it easy. When they die, their parts are recycled by your spleen into brand new blood. Your lips and mouth show the condition of your spleen.

Pancreas

Partially digested sugar and carbohydrates in the small intestine activate your pancreas, a fish-shaped organ with two jobs. Its first job is to produce and send out enzymes that break up sugar and carbohydrates into small pieces so they can be absorbed into the blood. The blood then carries the sugar to the cells, and the cells use the sugar as their main fuel to give the body energy. The pancreas' second job is to produce the hormone insulin.

What does insulin do and why do we need it? Your blood is the transport that carries oxygen and nutrients from your food to all the cells in your body. Each cell is a complete unit that needs energy to live. Sugar provides the fuel that keeps the cell working, much like gas in a car. Fats and proteins build and support the function of each cell. But how does that energy get inside? Digested proteins and fat enter cells easily. They have a key to the front door. But poor old sugar doesn't have a key. It needs a doorkeeper to let it in. This is what insulin is—it is the doorkeeper that allows sugar to enter a cell. If a cell does not have sugar to burn as fuel, then it will burn fat instead. That's why eliminating sugar from your diet will help you lose the fat that your body has stored for a rainy day. If you have no more fat to burn, then the hungry cells will look for another source of fuel. It is at this point that they start to use the protein inside of themselves, which is very harmful to your body.

Large Intestine & Urine Bladder

Your large intestine and urine bladder prepare and store solid and liquid waste for recycling—outside of your body.

Triple Heater

Your triple heater (never heard of it?) is not a physical organ, but rather an organ function. This one is a little tricky to explain. Remember the story about the teapot that I relayed to you in the introduction of this book? The triple heater is a good example of that story—different cultures observe the same thing from different viewpoints and then draw different conclusions. In Chinese medicine, harmony between the different organs is considered even more important than the health of each organ individually. The first phase of treatment is to harmonize the entire body and then focus on the affected organ. In contrast, Western medicine concentrates directly on curing the diseased organ.

So here's how the triple heater works: Imagine your trunk being divided into three sections. In the top section are your lungs and your heart. Breathing and purification of your blood happens here. In the middle section, digestion takes place in your stomach, liver, spleen, and pancreas. The lower part, below your navel, is where your kidneys, intestines, and reproductive organs are housed. This is the main recycling center, where the useful is separated from the useless and your personal waste is eliminated. The triple heater coordinates the functions of these three sections so that they all work together in harmony. It controls the temperature of the water in your cells, keeping everything at body temperature, the ideal level of warmth to keep things running smoothly.

From the Western point of view, the triple heater's job is done by your hormones and your autonomic nervous system—that is, all the things that keep on working without your having to do anything about it. Hormones are produced in your glands. If your body is a factory, then your glands are the managers. The general manager is your pituitary gland, situated right between your eyes, nestled within your brain. It is responsible for all the other glands, like the thyroid and adrenal glands, gonads, and so on. As your blood flows through the glands, it picks up instructions in the form of hormones. Hormones trigger specific organs into action. They are very potent; a little bit goes a long way. To know what is needed where, the general manager uses the world's most remarkable supercomputer—your brain.

Brain

Your brain is the center of consciousness, thought, intellect, and memory. It controls the functions of seeing, hearing, smelling, and speaking. The rich capillary system in your brain circulates a large amount of blood that provides a way of receiving and processing information about the other organs. Another communication system is the spinal marrow and nerves—your personal information superhighway.

Appendix

Your appendix looks like a little worm and is about as long as your index finger. Although it's "appended" to your intestines, it is part of your body's defense system, along with your tonsils and lymph nodes. Your appendix and tonsils are made of the same type of tissue and produce "defender" cells that seek, capture, and eliminate bacteria, viruses, and toxins, vagrants that have no place in a healthy body. Your tonsils are the first line of defense. They catch what they can before the enemy gets very far into your body. Your appendix catches toxins during digestion. Your spleen sends out cells that attack any bacteria, toxins, or viruses that manage to enter your bloodstream. The heat of this battle causes your temperature to rise.

Lymph Nodes

Your lymph nodes look like small bunches of grapes and are located around all your major organs and blood vessels. They provide a base for white blood cells to hang out until they are needed. The lymph nodes are involved in the first line of defense to stop the spread of infection in your body. If you cut your finger, the very first thing to react is your blood. White blood cells rush to the scene of the accident to fight off and kill bacteria. If they are not strong enough to do it alone or if the cut is very large and overwhelming, then the white cells e-mail a message to the lymph nodes under your arms to send reinforcements, ASAP.

The Whole Body

You can see how interdependent all these systems are. A weakness in one of them will cause a weakness in all the others. Of course, there is a lot more going on in your body than this, but I wanted to give you a simple overview of what your friends inside of you are busy doing, twenty-four hours a day, every day of your life. Take a look at the full body diagram on the previous page; notice how the organs fit snugly together—each is so very dependent upon the others. Because of this interconnectedness, all of the organs must be in harmony, with themselves and with each other, for an overall healthy and smooth-running system.

Some Potential Problems

First, I'd like to talk about diabetes. Diabetes is a condition that occurs when the pancreas cannot produce enough insulin to allow sugar to be absorbed into the cells. Some people have a genetic predisposition to develop diabetes. If these people don't pay attention to what they eat, there is a good chance that they will develop the disease. This is what happens: If a person with a genetic predisposition to diabetes eats sugar and sweet foods every day, then over the years, the insulin-producing cells in the pancreas that are already weak burn out and die from being overworked. When less insulin is produced, sugar cannot be absorbed into the cells and used for fuel. The sugar stays in the blood (you've probably heard of "high blood sugar"). Too much sugar in the blood corrodes the capillaries and, after a while, they become rigid and unable to do their job of absorbing nutrients and oxygen. Generally, after ten to fifteen years, people with unchecked diabetes will begin to have problems with their eyes, kidneys, and joints. These places have rich capillary systems that become damaged over time by too much sugar in the blood that flows through them.

People who have a family history of diabetes need to pay attention to the way they live. It is important that they avoid eating sugar or sweets and that they work in low-stress jobs. The onset of diabetes is preventable. If you feel thirsty all the time, have a dryness in your mouth, feel nervous, get "the shakes," and crave sugar, then you should get the situation checked out. Sugar cravings occur when cells are hungry for sugar. There could be plenty in your blood, but without insulin to unlock the door to the cell, they "hear it knocking, but it can't get in." If the condition has already developed, then medication is needed. In addition to the pre-scribed medication, eating the correct food and drink-ing a mixture of celery and parsley juice every day will help to counteract the high level of sugar in the blood.

Now, let's talk about another ailment. I'm sure you've all heard of gallstones, but do you know what they are or what causes them? If there are bacteria in the gall bladder, they can cause an infection that changes the quality of the bile. It gets sticky and acts like glue, sticking to the bacteria and dead cells. More and more of it accumulates and sticks. Eventually, many layers build up and create a "stone." These vary in quantity, shape, and size. They can be as tiny as a grain of sand or as large as a marble. The gall bladder is like a neat little pear-shaped sack. The stones irritate its inside walls, the "gall walls." They are sometimes pulled out of the gall bladder into the small intestine along with the normal bile flow and are eliminated. That's the good news. The bad news is that sometimes they get stuck in the bile duct (the little tube that connects the gall bladder to the small intestine). If this happens, the flow of bile is blocked. This leads to problems with digestion and causes a bile buildup in the gall bladder and liver, which makes the skin and the whites of the eyes take on a yellowish coloring and can cause a sharp pain just under the ribs on the right side of the body. In other words: big trouble!

If you have your gall bladder removed, your liver kindly takes over the job of sending bile into your intestine to let you digest fat. However, unlike the gall bladder, which squirts out a blast of bile when you need it most, the liver just lets it drip continuously, whether you need it or not. So, if you don't have a gall bladder, don't eat too much fat at once.

Bad Habits

Let's talk briefly about smoking. What about it? If you don't smoke, don't start. If you already smoke, one cigarette after lunch will not kill you. Nicotine stimulates your digestive juices, but if you smoke too much or smoke without eating, you will damage your stomach and lungs. Smoking will, in fact, damage all your systems because it creates an imbalance in your internal central heating system. So, if you cannot restrict yourself to one cigarette a day after a meal, it is better to quit—*soon*. If you do enjoy that cigarette after dinner, be aware that other people around you who don't smoke might not want to share it with you. Make a point never to smoke around babies or small children.

Now, let's move on to soft drinks. An often overlooked source of trouble in the West is the widespread consumption of carbonated drinks. We won't mention any names. Besides the fact that most carbonated drinks contain a huge amount of sugar (or equally unhealthy sugar substitute), the carbonation in the drink masquerades as digestive juice (and this includes carbonated water). This makes the real digestive juice producers in your body lazy. Your digestive system becomes dependent on carbonated drinks to do its job. It's all right to have a carbonated drink occasionally or when you need to bring up a burp—but not every day.

4

△△△△△△△△△△△△

A Tale of Two Headaches

Mary has a headache. Jane has a headache, too. They can both take two aspirins and call me in the morning. Maybe they'll feel better for a while, but chances are they will both call me back again next week complaining of another headache. Why?

Most headache medicines on the market may be effective pain relievers, but they do not address the *cause* of the headache. Until you identify and treat the cause, the problem will keep coming back to haunt you. Always remember, *not all headaches are created equal.*

First I'll tell you about Mary. Mary is in her forties. She's been getting headaches a couple of times a week for the last few months. When the headache begins, she gets very sensitive to noise and to light. She likes to be alone in a darkened room until the pain subsides.

She experiences a sharp pain that stretches from one eyebrow to the top of her ear on one side of her head. This kind of headache is commonly known as a migraine.

Mary is unhappy with her job. She is rather short-tempered and often has cravings for chocolate. From my experience, her symptoms indicate that the cause of her headaches is a problem with her digestion. This stems from an imbalance between her liver and gall bladder, caused by continuous stress in her lifestyle and eating the wrong foods.

What would I recommend to Mary? First of all, I would suggest that she change her diet. Nix the coffee, alcohol, nicotine, and hot spices. Forget about chocolate and sweets. When she craves chocolate she can make herself a morning cup of hot cocoa. (Mix one teaspoon of unsweetened cocoa powder and one teaspoon of honey into a quarter cup of hot milk. When the cocoa has dissolved, add more hot milk to fill the cup. Cocoa has lots of iron in it that supports the blood but none of the sugar and fat of chocolate.) Mary needs to eat more salads, green vegetables, and fresh fruit to harmonize her stomach and to obtain more minerals to strengthen her blood. Soups, salads, fresh dandelion greens, and fruit will calm her body and support the flow of energy in her liver. She would benefit from a cup of mint tea in the afternoon and before she goes to bed at night.

It would also be a good idea for her to find a job that she enjoys doing. Anger and frustration at spending time at a job you hate slowly builds up and poisons your liver.

Now let's meet Jane. Jane is in her sixties, retired, and has a calm disposition. When she gets a headache, she feels pain in the back of her head. It's worse when the weather starts to get cold. She often has aches and stiffness in her neck and shoulders, and sometimes feels a dull pain in her lower back. Jane complains of eyestrain when her headaches begin. She has an accumulation of cold in her body, a degenerative process (osteoporosis) in her vertebrae, and weak blood circulation in her upper back and neck. It is the weak circulation and accumulated cold that causes her headaches. Her problem is worse when the thermometer drops.

Jane needs hot drinks, especially cinnamon or ginger tea, to aid her digestion, promote the circulation of her blood, and warm up her body. She should eliminate cold foods like ice cream and iced drinks. She should avoid any extreme foods (see the seesaw in chapter 1). Rice and soup with a little spice added to them will warm her up. Jane should invest in a thermal scarf and make sure that her neck and back are kept toasty. A magnetic belt would do her a lot of good and a sauna would be beneficial to really warm up her toes. Light exercise, slow head rolls, stretching, yoga, and anything that develops flexibility in her back and neck will help Jane to avoid headaches in the future.

Here are a few more examples of common headaches and their origins.

Mike is a teenager. He's tall and gangly, sixteen years old, just got his driver's license, and can't wait to get on with his life. Like many teenagers, he's nervous, tense, and temperamental. His eating habits are bad: he prefers to hang out with his friends and grab some grub at the mall, he eats fast and washes down his food with lots of ice-cold cola, and he avoids eating home-cooked meals. Lately, headaches and stomachaches have been cramping his style; not only that, but he has to burp all the time and sometimes even vomits.

Mike's headaches and upset stomach usually hit right after he eats. Their source? Mike's weak stomach, which is due to his poor eating habits—both in style and content. First of all, Mike needs to *eat slowly*. He needs to eliminate cola, spicy food, fried foods, and, for the time being, meat. "Oh man!" I can hear him say, "What *can* I eat?" If Mike wants to eat at home, he can have lots of good food. He can start his day with a cup of licorice tea. For lunch and dinner, soup is great, accompanied by boiled foods, vegetables, yogurt, and fresh fruit. If Mike just can't break away from the gang, he can still find things to eat that will be better than what he was eating before. Many fast food places offer soup or salad—both good choices. He can also find a place that serves pasta with a nonspicy sauce, or eat vegetarian Chinese food. But he *cannot* drink cola.

I have already mentioned that carbonated drinks weaken the digestive system. In fact, drinking any liquid with food is not a good idea. Only "civilized" human beings drink water with their meals. Animals know to eat first and then drink. Maybe we can learn something from them. Drinking liquids with meals will dilute your digestive juices. You know what that means.

The main thing for Mike and for all of us to remember is to pay more attention to the food we eat—not just the kind of food but also how we eat it. When we read the paper or watch television while we eat, our brain disconnects from our stomach. Good digestion starts before we even begin to eat: We may see a delicious looking meal on television or smell good food cooking. These things produce saliva in our mouths, readying them for the intake of a meal. If you don't pay attention to the food you are eating or if you eat food that is unappetizing, then your body produces less digestive juice and you can develop a "lazy stomach," leading to problems with your digestion. *Fast food = fast death.*

Mike needs to watch his diet very carefully for a couple of weeks. After that, yogurt and cereal will start his day off well. Fresh fruit in his pocket and fresh vegetables for lunch will keep him on the right track. He can start to eat meat again and have the occasional junk food meal and cola. But if he reverts to his previous way of eating, his headaches will return.

Meet Mike's Auntie Agnes. Agnes feels a dull pain all over her head. She's thirty years old and works as a secretary. Mike says, "Auntie Agnes always moves in slow motion." He thinks it's funny. Agnes doesn't. She's overweight, has a pale complexion, feels tired all the time, and has no energy. She doesn't like to walk, to exercise, or to do anything physical. She gets up in the morning and goes through her day like a zombie. She has no hopes or dreams and is not in a relationship. Every day she takes the bus to work. She always feels a dull ache in her head that gets worse in the afternoon. She often falls asleep in the bus on her way home and wakes up feeling worse. Poor Agnes. She's a mess!

Agnes's headache is caused by a lack of life force. The dull pain in her head comes from dullness in her whole body. She needs to recharge her blood and increase the circulation of blood in her body. To put it in the poetic terms of Chinese imagery: the energy in her body has pooled into a stagnant lake rather than a flowing river.

Agnes needs to shake herself by the shoulders and make some changes in her lifestyle. The first thing that she needs to do is *move*. Instead of taking the bus all the way to work she can get off one block earlier and walk the rest of the way. In the evening she can do the same thing on her way home. When that becomes comfortable then she can get off two blocks earlier.

At work she can nibble on healthy snacks like strawberries, raspberries, or blackberries rather than eating candy or potato chips. Instead of coffee she can have fresh orange or carrot juice. A cup of stimulating cinnamon or ginger tea in the morning, and mint tea in the afternoon and evening will help balance Agnes' system. Agnes must forget about junk food, caffeine, nicotine, chocolate, and sodas. When she starts to feel more alive, she can find something she likes to do that will provide both exercise and social contact, such as taking a dance class or playing softball every weekend.

Let's meet one more lady. Her name is Sally. She doesn't get headaches very often and usually feels pretty good. She leads an active life, eats well, and has a well-paying job that she loves. She's happily married with two lovely children and she finds time to go to her aerobics class twice a week. She's a Super Mom, and has everything "under control." Today, though, Sally has a headache. She noticed that when she gets a headache, it's often just before her menstrual period starts. The pain throbs in her temples. This kind of headache is like a little wake-up call. It says, "Hey! Slow down and take care of your body!" What Sally needs is *rest*. It's time to tell the family, "Excuse me, but I need to take care of *myself* now." A hot bath with a few drops of lavender oil, relaxing music, and a cup of mint, chamomile, or valerian tea will calm her body, relax her muscles, and regulate her sleep. Sally needs to put on the brakes. Her body needs time to renew and refresh itself.

It used to be that a woman would take to her couch when she had her menstrual period; it's a time that nature sets aside for women to refresh and renew their energy. These days, women don't have the luxury of quietly staying at home during menstruation. Women, if you are aware that nature requires a little quiet time, then make a gesture to accommodate it. Make a date with yourself to spend at least one quiet evening at home per month. Ask the family's indulgence. Don't answer the phone. Don't bring work home. For one night a month, just pamper yourself. Think of it as an investment in health.

Getting back to our headaches: Did you know that 80 percent of headaches are symptoms of a functional imbalance either between organs or between the body and its environment? When you are suffering from a headache, by all means take an aspirin or a mild painkiller, but when the pain subsides, don't just sit and wait for the next attack. Fight back! Start to make changes in your lifestyle and diet. If you smoke, quit. Walk, or start an exercise program. Tall orders, I know, but your life is at stake. Acupuncture can help a lot to ease the discomfort of transition to a healthier lifestyle. It tunes your body and helps to support the weaknesses that make change difficult. I'll tell you more about how acupuncture works in chapter 8.

If headaches still persist even after you have improved your lifestyle, it is time to have a checkup to see if there is a localized, specific problem of the sinus, ears, eyes, nose, or teeth, genetic damage of blood vessels, a tumor, or something else. If you have already made changes toward a healthier lifestyle, your body will be in a much stronger position to tackle a more serious problem if that proves to be the cause of your pain.

5

▲▲▲▲▲▲▲▲▲▲▲

Show Some Emotion

Someone said, "We are what we eat," but that's not enough. Descartes said, "I think, therefore I am," but that is not complete. The philosopher John Donne said, "No man is an island." Now that's getting closer. We are all part of a greater whole. We experience our environment through our *feelings*; through the feeling of our five senses: sight, sound, taste, touch, and smell; through the feelings perceived as emotions; and through hunches and insights, which are a sort of mental feeling.

All contact with our environment has an influence on our health. Without our five senses we would have no knowledge of the world around us. They allow us to interact with our environment and to survive and enjoy life. Our hunches and instincts also help us to survive, if we pay attention to them. People who live close to nature have more sensitive senses and keener perception. They are aware of the subtle changes of temperature and of the behavior of birds and animals. They have to be. Their survival depends on it.

As we became more technologically advanced, we learned to control our immediate environment. We live in comfortable houses with heating and cooling systems. Our food comes from the grocery store, rather than from hunting and gathering. All of this gives us more time for other things, like developing arts and technology or watching TV.

However, our survival still depends on our interaction with the world through the food we eat, the air we breathe, and the relationships we form. As well as getting information about our physical environment, we also get information about the other people who share it with us. This brings me to the next piece of the puzzle of total health: *emotions*!

Do you know the difference between a feeling and an emotion? A feeling is what you actually experience. Feelings show in your body. For example, if you get angry, your face might flush and your fists might clench; you might feel tension in your jaw. You know you're angry. The emotion that goes with that feeling is more complicated: it involves a judgment about that feeling; a judgment that is usually based on past experiences of feeling angry. Your reactions to the emotion of anger can be very disproportional to the situation at hand, the event that produced the feeling of anger. It's important to observe how you react when faced with a strong feeling or emotion. In order to stay healthy, it's good to learn the trick of acknowledging your feelings without getting carried away by the emotion. It takes some practice, to be sure, but the first step is realizing the difference.

Think of feelings as the strings of a guitar and emotions as the sound that comes out when they are strummed. The sound depends on how tight the strings are. If they are too tight then the sound is hard. If they are too loose then the sound is weak. The trick is to have the strings at just the right tension and tuned in relationship to one another so the resulting sound is harmonious.

As you can see from this example, feelings and emotions take on physical form in your body. Continuous strong emotions directly affect the different organs in your body. On the following page is a chart that shows some of the correspondences (Chinese style) between organs, emotions, and other interesting things that you might not have known were related to one another.

Yin Organ	Yang Organ	Feature	Season	Emotion	Body Link	Energy	Taste	Element
Liver	Gall Bladder	Eyes	Spring	Anger	Skin & Hair	Dry	Sour	Metal
Heart	Small Intestine	Tongue	Summer	Happiness Unhappiness	Bones	Cold	Spicy	Water
Lungs	Large Intestine	Nose	Autumn	Sadness	Blood Vessels	Heat	Pungent	Fire
Kidney	Urine Bladder	Ear	Winter	Fear	Muscles	Wind	Salty	Wood
Stomach	Spleen	Lips	The end of each season	Nervousness Worry	Complexion	Damp	Sweet	Earth

Sadness affects your lungs. Think of all the nineteenth-century stories in which the star-crossed lover expires from tuberculosis. Lungs are paired with the large intestines. Sadness can cause a blockage of energy in them, a sluggishness that leads to constipation. If sadness is a part of your life, take a walk in nature, breathe deeply, listen to the birds singing, and know that the sadness will pass.

Anger affects your liver and gall bladder. In my language, we have the expression, "I was so angry, I vomited bile." In English, you say, "I was so angry I saw red." The eyes, you remember, are associated with the liver.

When you are feeling angry, stop and take a breath. Observe where you are holding the anger in your body. In your fists? In your jaw? Try to relax your body when you exhale. If you have a buildup of unexpressed anger, find a place where you can *yell*. Go to a local sporting event or to a noisy highway and yell until you feel the anger releasing. Singing is another good way to relieve a buildup of anger. Join a choir. Let go with a scream or a song while you're driving (if you don't have a convertible, that is). Just remember to keep your eyes open.

Joy! What's wrong with that? How can we have too much joy? Well, let's say you've just heard about the birth of your first grandchild or that you won $64 million in the lottery. A pleasant shock, but a shock nonetheless. If your heart is weak, you may spend all your winnings on doctor's bills. Too much of a good thing can weaken your heart and your small intestine. What to do? Relax and *exhale!* Joy is wonderful, but sometimes if you laugh too much it's hard to catch your breath. So remember to exhale.

Nervousness and worry affect your spleen and stomach. This is a very common condition in modern life. You worry about survival and about how to make ends meet; you get nervous in traffic; you have stress in your daily life. All of this creates an imbalance in your stomach. This imbalance sometimes causes overeating, cravings for the wrong food, or a lack of appetite. You can get caught up in a downward spiral of stomach problems. What to do? Change your habits or your job, if you can. Find work you enjoy and a mode of transportation that doesn't cause stress. Avoid eating hot or spicy foods and smoking. Try to eat at regular times and don't eat heavy food late in the evening. Make time to spend with your friends. Learn and practice anti-stress techniques such as deep breathing, meditation, or yoga. Relax, man.

Fear. This is a big one. Babies who are startled will wet their pants. This is a natural reaction because fear directly affects the kidney and urine bladder. Adults learn to control and suppress this natural reaction.

Thank goodness. But we don't learn what we can do to prevent a buildup of fear in our bodies. Fear is the deepest held emotion. It is the strongest and the most subtle. The "fight or flight" response is programmed into us. In today's society, we must curb our natural instincts; feelings of fear get stuck and are held in our bodies.

The best we can do is to become *aware* of the fear that we are holding. It runs deep in our subconscious. Think of insurance. The whole concept is based on our fear that something awful is going to happen and we must somehow be "covered." When we watch the news, we see all the worst that society and nature have to offer. Good news is not news. Think about it. We are treated to stories of murder, rape, accidents, and natural disasters. All of this makes us fearful that something like that can happen to us. Our brains switch off for a moment and we forget that the chances of something like that happening to us are, in reality, pretty slim. We need to keep a sense of perspective and rational thinking while being bombarded with all this negative information.

I'm not suggesting you live recklessly or take unnecessary chances, but *don't let fear paralyze you.* A lot of it is in our imagination. Learn to moderate it. Turn off the television or limit your viewing to programs on animals and see how they cope with life in the wild. Getting on top of fear is all about awareness. Respect the difficulties in your life and accept them, but see them for what they are, not for what they may become.

Remember, you don't experience one emotion at a time. Generally, you are presented with a lovely bouquet of emotions. Sometimes it's hard to realize exactly what it is that you are feeling. That's when it's good to have a look at what's going on inside of your body for *clues.*

Emotions can lead to serious mental and physical problems if they are extreme and continuous and allowed to build up over time. Find moderation in your emotions. If your lifestyle is amiss, you will find yourself in extreme situations that will eventually manifest in your physical body and destroy your health.

Spend more time doing what you like to do, what makes you happy. If you can't change your job right away, then make time for a hobby that you enjoy. Spend time with people you like and who share your interests. Being healthy includes having good company, pleasant times, and humor.

Imagine that you have an emotion quota. Imagine that any emotion can fill it up. So, why not fill it with happiness and pleasure? You'll find that there is less room for sadness, anger, and fear. It's your choice, you know. In the immortal words of Bobbie McFerrin, "Don't worry, be happy."

6

△△△△△△△△△△△

What You Can't See
Can Hurt You

ow that you understand Yin and Yang and have had a look at what's going on inside of you, I'd like to spend some time explaining what is going on outside of you, energetically, that can affect your health. And that is *plenty*.

One hundred years ago, a television set would have been unimaginable. Now we take for granted that someone miles away can be seen right in front of us on our television screen. How about the magic of the remote control? Click, click, and something happens to the television, apparently all by itself. Cellular phones extend the reach of your voice without any cords or wires. I think we all know that this "magic" is actually a physical phenomenon (something we learned about in physics class but have now totally forgotten). The point is, we can't see anything but we know something is there.

It's common knowledge that there are a lot of stray waves constantly flying through the air that are created by televisions, radios, microwaves, computers, cell phones, radars, and powerful emissions from high-tension wires and high-voltage power stations, for example.

These waves vibrate over a wide spectrum of frequencies. How do all the different waves affect us? Extensive research is being conducted in Europe, Japan, and the United States to find out. Over the last few decades, as more and more technical equipment is being developed and widely used, there is a growing concern about their health consequences. People know from experience that exposure to these waves weaken their system. Now it's up to the scientists to explain why.

Less well-known are the subtle vibrations that are under our feet; some are manmade and others occur naturally.

Our earth is a giant magnet. Its rotation produces electrical currents in the earth's molten metal core. These electromagnetic currents create subtle, invisible vibrations that are everywhere—in the earth itself, in the air, in us, and in every living thing. Life on earth evolved in accordance with these subtle but ever-present vibrations. All life is dependent on them to regulate the subtle vibrations within.

Imagine a grid of energetic "walls" about eight inches wide that run north to south and east to west all around the globe.

The *real* World Wide Web:

The ones running north to south are about six feet apart. The ones that run east to west are a little closer together. You can find these walls everywhere.

They can be disturbing to humans. If you spend a lot of time exposed to them, you may feel *tense, tired, or weak*. Cats, on the other hand, really enjoy the energy that comes from these places. They seem to feel a comfortable warmth in there. Strange but true. So, don't sleep where your cat sleeps.

If the walls are uncomfortable, then the spots where they cross are a pain. This is how they work.

Each line has a charge, either positive or negative.

Where positive and negative lines cross, the effect is minimal.

However, on the spots where there is a double charge, either positive or negative, there's a double whammy.

These hot spots are known in the trade as Hartmann Knots, after Dr. Ernst Hartmann, who made this discovery. Following is an example of what a Hartmann Knot can do.

Mr. and Mrs. Smith are a young couple who used to be happily married, but lately there's been trouble in paradise. Mrs. Smith wakes up feeling tired every morning. She tosses and turns all night and the movement bothers Mr. Smith. To top it all off, the light has gone out of their love life. Everything was fine until they moved into their new house a few months ago, but everything's been going downhill since. Why? Let's have a look at the invisible walls in the Smiths' new bedroom and see what's happening.

Mrs. Smith sleeps on an energetic wall. There is no way that she can have a good night's sleep there. She twists and turns all night, disturbing Mr. Smith. Look at the location of the other line. No wonder they never feel "in the mood" anymore. Every morning she hits the snooze button one, two, three times. When she finally crawls out of bed, she needs two cups of coffee just to open her eyes. If Mrs. Smith continues to sleep in this place, chances are she will develop a problem in her abdomen, womb, or lower back because two walls cross right at that spot. The good news for this couple is that they can move their bed to a place that is not influenced by energetic walls and they will probably feel like popping open a bottle of champagne in a week or two. Pretty simple.

Here's another example.

George is a nice guy who is successful at his job and popular with his colleagues. But since he moved into his new apartment, his temper had been short and he complains of terrible headaches. Let's see why.

You guessed it. All night George's head is in a Hartmann Knot. No matter what he does to strengthen his energy in the daytime, every night it drains out again because of the harmful vibrations in this spot.

Another factor that contributes to George's headache is the presence of electromagnetic fields that are emitted from his alarm clock, cell phone charger, and bedside lamp. Yes, these things are useful and generally not harmful, but they should not be placed next to George's head. Do you have a clock, radio, telephone, extension cord, lamp, or other electrical appliance near your head, like George? Move them farther away! Throw away your electric blanket. They produce electromagnetic fields when you turn them on. Even when they are turned off, the wires in them amplify any disturbing vibrations that may be around you. Down comforters will keep you warmer with none of the side effects (and you'll have lower electricity bills, too).

It is not yet known whether these vibrational walls originate in the earth or if they come from space, pulled in by the earth's gravity and reflected back. Maybe they are caused by the interaction between the earth and cosmic rays. I don't know. I do know the effect they have. In the past, I found that sometimes after I treated a patient by balancing their energy with acupuncture, correct food, medicinal herbs—doing everything that I knew should have made them feel better—they would leave my place feeling great but come back in a day or two with no energy. We built up his energy by day but he lost it by night. I knew I was giving the right treatment and could see that the energy was much stronger after a treatment, so what was happening? Time and time again, I went to check where the patient spent his time. Guess what I found? That's right. Bad vibes! Move the bed and, voilá, no more energy leaking and the patient's health took a turn for the better. I learned from experience that eliminating harmful vibrations from personal surroundings is a very important piece in the puzzle of total health.

As if a World Wide Web of disturbing vibrations is not enough, there are other types of subtle vibrations that are even worse. These include mineral deposits, caves, natural faults in the earth, and, most commonly, underground streams, either flowing naturally or in pipes.

This is what happens with underground water: Imagine a river. A river flows. It flows in a particular direction. As the water flows through the pipe (either manmade or a natural tunnel), it creates turbulent circulation.

This is how it works in an enclosed system. It's a good idea to make note of this because it's very important information. But *why* is this information so significant? What's going on there? Well, when water moves like this, it creates friction. Friction causes vibrations that travel and expand. To give you an example, think of a stone that is dropped into a calm pond. The waves travel slowly out from the center, right? Well, these vibrations behave in a similar way, only in three dimensions. Check out the illustrations on the following pages—perhaps you'll get a better understanding of how this works.

Look what happens!

These are normal vibrations of the earth:

Here's an underground stream. The waves from the running water deviate the normal vibrations, causing us to lose our vital connection with Mother Earth.

As you can see, that one little stream can affect a wide area.

Look at the apartment house next door. The lower floors are unaffected by the underground stream, but the upper floors catch it!

Some time ago, a friend planned to build a house and asked me to check the lot for him. At the time, he was using the piece of land to graze horses. I found an underground stream running right through the place he planned to build his house. I asked the man who tended the horses if the horses liked to spend their time in the shady place near their watering trough. He told me, "Oh, no. They come and drink and then go over there." He indicated another area on the far side of the property. The trough was fed by a spring. The area around it was influenced by an underground stream that disturbed the horses.

Like the horses, experienced dowsers are able to locate the presence of underground water. It's great to find water for a well or for irrigation but it's not so good to build a house above an underground stream. What happens? You know that your body is about 70 percent water, right? The strong vibrations caused by movement of the underground water affect the water in your body. Your own personal water starts to feel a connection with the outside vibrations. Imagine that you hear loud music playing. Your foot starts tapping in time to the rhythm. You can't help it. The water in your body can't help it either. These vibrations are great for the underground water but not for your water. When you want to have a good night's sleep, the water in your body is busy partying. How do you know if your bed is over underground vibrations? Easy. You continually wake up feeling tired, like you've been partying all night, too.

Just to make matters worse, if you live or work in a tall building that has a lot of metal reinforcement in it, guess what happens? The metal in the structure of the building amplifies all vibrations and you get a double dose.

A friend of mine lives in a big house with four bedrooms and a lovely view of the sea. Both she and her son were feeling down so I offered to give them a checkup at their home. When I stepped into the house I felt very uncomfortable. I sensed a slight pressure in my head when I walked through the door. Through my research and experience, I have become more aware of and sensitive to the presence of vibrations. My friend has three big dogs. She told me that all the dogs slept in one corner of the house. It was funny to see three large dogs curled up together in one corner. When I checked the house for underground vibrations, I found that the only good spot in the house was the corner where the dogs slept. So, watch your dogs. Their bodies react to the presence of vibrations much like ours. They naturally go to the places that are good for us. Draw the line, though, at sleeping in the doghouse.

In the past, when people lived closer to nature, they knew these things. They would watch the animals and birds and learn from them. People were nomadic and followed animals. They watched where the animals liked to hang out and would then pitch their tents there. Today, we suffer because we have forgotten this knowledge.

So, what to do? First of all, if you are not getting a good night's sleep, *move your bed.* With a little practice with dowsing rods or the muscle test (see appendix B), you can find out where the harmful spots are. Ideally, it's best to be in a clear spot with your head to the north and your feet to the south, following the flow of the earth's magnetic field. Second best is with your head to east and your feet to the west. That way you will be aligned with the rotational force of the earth. However, it's better to be any-which-way in a spot that is clear of disturbing vibrations then correctly aligned in a harmful spot.

Watch your plants. Most plants do not like places with strong vibrations. They cannot be healthy if they are exposed to them. More than likely, a person with a green thumb is someone who lives in a place that is not affected by harmful vibrations.

If you have nowhere to move your bed, there are some things that you can do to protect yourself. I'll get to that later in the next chapter.

Another important source of disturbance are electromagnetic fields. Many creatures depend on the natural geomagnetic fields that they use as pathways to guide them on their seasonal migrations. Birds have a center in their brains that responds to magnetic fields.

The magnetic field varies in intensity depending on the seasons and the time of day. This is Cosmic Law and all organisms are a part of it—including us. Birds have a center in their brains that responds to magnetic fields. All living beings respond to natural electromagnetic fields to help them to survive. Humans do, too, but we've forgotten how it works.

Over the last century, there have been incredible technological developments: electricity, radio, television, household appliances, microwave ovens, personal computers, cell phones, and so forth. All these things create new fields that are different in frequency from those in nature, both in quality and quantity.

What effect do these electromagnetic fields have on the body? Imagine a healthy body as an orchestra with all the parts, the organs and the cells playing together in the same rhythm and producing a harmonious sound. Now imagine a loud drum outside the concert hall beating at a different rhythm. After a while, the weakest member of the orchestra will pick up the rhythm of the drum. This player throws off the whole orchestra and pretty soon the sound is no longer harmonious.

A healthy body tries to keep its own rhythm—optimum health—but if it is continually exposed to harmful vibrations in the environment, it cannot stick to its own rhythm and slowly loses the game on all levels. It is very important to understand the duration, quality, and quantity of exposure to harmful electromagnetic fields.

What to do? If you have high voltage power lines running above your house or if you live close to a power plant or transformer, *move.* If you have lamps, clocks, extension cords, televisions, or radios near your bed, *move them.* Just do it. As you can imagine, spending many hours in front of a computer is not very good for you. Make sure that you sit a good distance from the screen and take frequent breaks to stretch and get some fresh air to revive your energy. Protect yourself with an electromagnetic field neutralizer or put an amethyst cluster between you and the computer. I'll tell you why in the next chapter.

7

△△△△△△△△△△

Rock and Roll

I'd now like to tell you some interesting things about rocks. Well, not exactly rocks . . . this chapter is about crystals, gemstones, and magnets, and how you can use them to improve your health and well-being.

They say a diamond is a girl's best friend. Why? Why do you think diamonds are prized beyond any other stone? Maybe ancient people knew more than we give them credit for. It has to do with light. A diamond is so precious because all the colors of the spectrum are contained in it.

Light works in a funny way. Sunlight contains all the colors of the rainbow. A rainbow happens simply because water vapor in the air breaks light up into its parts. Do you remember the seven colors of the rainbow? They are red, orange, yellow, green, blue, indigo, and violet. Together these colors make white light.

It's very pretty, but what does this have to do with my health? To be healthy is to be whole, to be complete, to have all your systems working optimally together. It's like white light—a total whole spectrum in balance with itself.

We see different colors because each one is vibrating at a different frequency. Parts of us vibrate at different frequencies, too. The trick for achieving good health is to get our whole body to vibrate in *harmony*. The subtle forms of healing like aromatherapy, flower essences, and sound and color therapy all work to increase our life force and bring our bodies into optimum balance. Once we are balanced on the etheric level, good health can begin to come to the physical level, too.

Acupuncture works somewhere in between the physical and etheric bodies. It regulates the flow of energy in the body to increase vitality. Using hair-fine needles to stimulate particular points along energetic highways and byways, acupuncture strengthens and balances the life force, which in turn allows the body's own natural healing to occur. That's why acupuncture has no negative side effects; the body heals itself.

We talked before about balancing the Yin and Yang energy in your body. We saw how all the organs are interdependent. Now I'll show you another system that has only recently been brought to the attention of the West, though it has been common knowledge in Eastern cultures for thousands of years.

Do you know about your chakras? Every body has seven major chakras. Each is a center of energy; a wheel of light spinning like a whirlpool. They are outward projections of your state of health. Each one relates to a different aspect of your physical, emotional, and mental well-being. Each one is also associated with a color and a particular organ. Now I want to introduce you to the colors and the chakras.

Within the rainbow, there are two main divisions of color: the warm colors of the red spectrum (Yang), and the cool colors of the blue spectrum (Yin). All colors are represented in the human body; the warm colors are lower down and the cool colors are up above; green, the color of nature, is right in the middle.

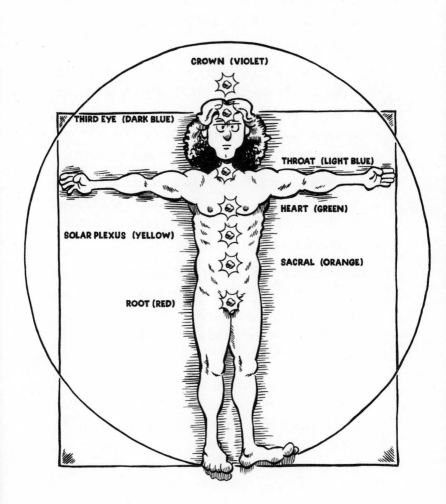

The First Chakra (Root) is at the base of your spine. It relates to your life force, survival, strength, and power. Its color is red and its gemstones are ruby, jasper, and coral.

The Second Chakra (Sacral) is in the center of your abdomen, about a hand's width below your navel. It relates to physical energy, sexuality, romantic love, and your reproductive organs. Its color is orange and its gemstones are carnelian, tiger-eye, and amber.

The Third Chakra (Solar Plexus) is just above your navel. It relates to digestion, mental functions, and control of the physical body. Its color is yellow and its gemstones are citrine and yellow topaz.

The Fourth Chakra (Heart) is in the center of your chest. It relates to emotions, feelings, and the functions of the heart and lungs, circulation and respiration. Its color is green and its gemstones are emerald, jade, and malachite.

The Fifth Chakra (Throat) is at your throat. It relates to communication and expression. It's connected to the tongue, larynx, pharynx, and thyroid gland. Its color is light blue and its gemstones are turquoise, lapis lazuli, and sapphire.

The Sixth Chakra (Third Eye) is in the center of your forehead. It relates to intuition and perception. It is connected to the pineal gland and to your senses of sight, smell, and hearing. Its color is indigo and its gemstones are sapphire, blue agate, and aquamarine.

The Seventh Chakra (Crown) is on the top of your head. It is your connection to the Divine. Its color is violet and its gemstone is amethyst.

I'm presenting this very basic information about chakras so I can go on and give you some practical tips about using stones. There are many good books that can give you detailed information about the chakras. Take a look at the bibliography at the end of this book.

Stones Are Your Friends

One of the most user-friendly stones that I've discovered is the quartz crystal. Quartz is related to the diamond in that they are both colorless (since they are, in essence, all colors) and carry the full spectrum of vibrations of light. Place a diamond or a quartz crystal in the sun and you can see all the colors of the rainbow. The clearer the stone, the brighter the colors. Quartz crystals are either clear or cloudy. The clear ones carry Yang energy and the cloudy ones carry Yin energy. You can use pieces of quartz to help get yourself in balance.

For example, if you are feeling low (Yin), hold or wear a clear quartz crystal or meditate while looking at one. You can also put a clear quartz crystal in a glass of spring water. Leave it there overnight. In the morning, remove the stone and drink the water. The presence of the clear quartz crystal "Yangizes" the water and you will feel revitalized if you continually drink "crystallized" water over a period of two to three weeks. Don't drink it at bedtime, though—it might keep you awake.

Here is a little secret for people who love to drink wine but don't like the way they feel the morning after. Place a clear quartz crystal (about the size of your thumb) in your wine before you drink it. Leave it in for about three to five minutes for a glass of wine, and about twenty minutes for a bottle. Not only will the wine taste much mellower, but you won't feel such strong effects. Why? We saw before that alcohol is Yin. By bringing it in contact with a Yang stone, the extreme Yin is brought into balance, moving closer to the center of the seesaw. This gives a whole new meaning to a drink "on the rocks."

I've done exhaustive research on this subject and have enjoyed every delicious moment of it. One of my favorite experiments is to pour one glass of wine from the bottle, put a crystal in the remainder, and wait a while. I then offer a glass of the "crystal" wine to my friends and ask them to compare it to the "control" glass that I poured earlier. I experimented on a friend who considers himself a wine connoisseur. He took the first glass, the crystal wine. Carefully, he swirled it around in the glass and delicately sniffed its bouquet. Tasting it, he proclaimed, "A delightful little wine . . . full bodied and mellow, with just a hint of blackcurrant." I gave him the second glass, the control glass. He nearly spat out the wine. "You don't expect me to drink this!" I loved the look on his face when I told him that it was from the same bottle. To this day I'm not sure he believed me. Don't take my word that this works—try it yourself.

The ancient people knew this trick. They placed amethyst crystals in their wine barrels. After some time, the amethyst moderated the strong Yin energy of the wine and mellowed it. In fact, amethyst is a Greek word that literally means "not intoxicated."

Another revitalizing technique is to get two quartz crystals, one clear and one cloudy. Men and women have to do this exercise differently. Why? Let me explain: A human is like a magnet with two poles. In a man, energy spirals from the sky toward the earth; in a woman, energy spirals from the earth to the sky.

Now for the exercise.

Sit comfortably. Make sure that you are not wearing tight clothing or shoes. Remove your jewelry. Ladies first: Hold the clear quartz in your left hand with the point facing away from you. Hold the cloudy stone in your right hand with the point facing toward you. Gentlemen, you hold the stones the opposite way: Hold the clear stone in your right hand with the point facing outward and the cloudy stone in your left hand with the point facing toward you. You'll be able to feel a light electrical current passing through your arms, heart, and shoulders. This little current can accelerate your energy flow and help dissolve blockages in your system. Try it and see. I find that it also intensifies my meditation.

Have you ever given any thought as to why kings and queens of old wore jeweled crowns? To make them seem taller and more imposing? Maybe. But could there be another reason? Rulers need a clear head to make decisions that are a matter of life or death to their people, or themselves. The metal of their crowns and the use of precious stones supported their subtle energy. Their energetic flow was stimulated and their power of perception sharpened. The Old Testament of the Bible gives very specific instructions for making a jeweled breastplate for Aaron, the brother of Moses (Exodus 28:17–21). There is a legend that Alexander the Great's conquest of the world was halted after he received a gift of a jeweled crown from the existing rulers of a province in India. I believe that the crown was specially designed to cause the devastating headache that led to Alexander's demise.

Many books have been written about the healing properties of crystals and gemstones. Again, I'll ask you to look at the bibliography. I promised a simple book, so I'll just give you a few more tried and true tips about our friends from the mineral kingdom.

Feel a sore throat (a Yang problem) coming on? Try a turquoise (a Yin stone). Turquoise is a light blue stone. It relates to the throat chakra. You can hang a turquoise on a short chain so it rests in the little hollow at the base of your neck; or tape a small stone to the same spot with medical tape. If you do this at the first sign of a sore throat, chances are you won't have a second sign.

For menstrual cramps or indigestion (Yin problems), try taping a carnelian (a Yang stone) to your tummy. A carnelian is a slightly translucent orange-colored stone. I know it looks strange, but the energy of the stone supports and balances your second chakra, which will make you feel a whole lot better.

On a summer day (Yang), when you're feeling hot already, it's best not to wear gold jewelry or amber (they are also Yang). Wearing these will make you feel even warmer. Wear them when it is cold to warm you up. Silver (Yin) has the opposite effect.

An amethyst will help protect you from the effects of strong vibrations in your environment. Wear one next to your body for protection. It's a good idea to place an amethyst cluster between you and your computer so that the energy of the stone strengthens your subtle energy, making you less vulnerable to the harmful effects of the strong electromagnetic vibrations coming out of the computer.

If you cannot move your bed or workplace, you can put amethyst clusters or slices of agate (four to five inches in diameter) underneath your bed or the chair you work in. This will dissipate strong underground vibrations. In the case of your bed, you will need enough stones to protect its entire area. The stones must be placed under the mattress in such a way that there are no energetic gaps. One amethyst cluster about the size of your fist will protect about two square feet of space. A single bed will need about three stones. If there is space left unprotected, the vibrations may be concentrated in one area of your body.

To make sure you've got it all covered, sit on the bed and try the muscle test (see appendix B).

Getting back to where we started: A diamond will strengthen and protect your entire aura. So, a diamond really can be seen as a girl's best friend—and a boy's, too.

We have discussed a stone that is full of light, the diamond; now let's have a look at a very dark one, a lodestone, more commonly known as a magnet. Do you remember playing with magnets as a child? I do. I was fascinated with how they stuck to one another for no apparent reason. I turned one around and felt them pushing each other apart, but no matter how hard and long I tried, I couldn't push them together. Why not? What was this invisible force that pulled the magnets together or kept them apart? Why and what, again!

The mysterious force is magnetism. The earth, as I mentioned before, is a huge magnet. Each small magnet works in the same way as the earth does. Every individual magnet has its own north and south poles. The north pole pushes out and the south pole pulls in. When two magnets are near one another and can move freely, their north and south poles will naturally join together. But try to put the two north poles or the two south poles together. Not only will they refuse to stick together, but they will push each other apart. Why? In the case of two north (pushing out) poles, their force pushes each other apart. In the case of the south (pulling in) poles, each one's energy is contracted; there is nothing for the other to pull. The moral of this story: Opposites attract!

Of all the wonders of the mineral kingdom, magnets are unique. They are the only stones that have their own electromagnet charge. Within their structure, they have both positively and negatively charged particles (Yin and Yang). In each individual magnet, the charge flows in one direction, from one end to the other. When it meets another magnet, it will turn itself in such a way that the flow will continue into its neighbor. For two to be drawn together, it is necessary to have a force that attracts and a force that repels. No matter how hard we try to connect similar ends together, those invisible but powerful energies won't let us do it.

In a healthy body, there is a dynamic balance of positive and negative particles. Through our everyday activities we use an uneven amount of them. Every cell in your body needs to replace the particles that have been used up in order to regain its balance and do its job. That's where magnets come in. Using magnets as a therapeutic tool supports our busy cells and makes us feel good. The stones I mentioned earlier in this chapter work gently to balance your mental and emotional energy, allowing your physical body to heal itself. A magnet's energy works from the opposite direction, penetrating and stimulating the physical body directly, supporting tissues, fluids, and organs on the cellular level and speeding the healing process. Once your body feel better, you relax and your mind and emotions become more balanced as well.

Magnets are being used more frequently to diagnose and treat diseases. Magnetic Resonance Imaging (MRI) has made it possible to see inside the human body in a way that was not possible in the past. Magnets are also used in some delicate surgeries. Experienced magnetotherapists successfully treat acute and chronic diseases as diverse as asthma, paralysis, and even cancer in its early stages.

There are many magnetic products on the market. These magnets are not original lodestones but man-made material that has the same magnetic properties. These products are handy to have around. Magnetic insoles can give you a lift. A magnetic mattress can help with insomnia. Therapeutic magnets placed next to injuries will help them heal. Even refrigerator magnets can make bruises disappear faster.

Magnets are particularly effective to treat rheumatism, which is the result of an excess of Yin, an accumulation of cold in the joints and muscles. There is a lack of circulation and a blockage in the free flow of energy, which causes pain and sometimes swelling. Magnets, correctly applied to the joints, work to unblock the stagnant energy and promote circulation, allowing fresh blood to carry the accumulated toxins away. I'll explain more about how your internal energy works in the next chapter.

8

△△△△△△△△△△△△

Say "Chee"

Chi (pronounced "chee"), ki, prana—many different names for the same thing: life force. Chi is the life force that flows through your body like a river, all the time, from the moment you are conceived until your last cell dies. The existence of chi is only now beginning to be known and accepted in the Western world. Oriental martial arts were introduced to the West a few decades ago. Martial arts work by strengthening a person's chi, and chi is in the name of many styles of martial arts—Chi Gong, Tai Chi, aikido, and so forth. They also train a person to achieve greater sensitivity to the energy both inside of them and around them. In that way, they are able to anticipate their opponent's move as if "by magic" and take action before the blow reaches them.

Acupuncture works with the flow of chi in your body. Imagine a river flowing freely to the sea. Picture a busy little beaver building a dam in its stream. The water cannot flow down to the valley as before and the plants in the valley start to wither and die. The chi flow in your body works the same way. If your chi is blocked, then the life force is prevented from flowing freely and after some time, physical symptoms will begin to appear in your body. That's why acupuncture works so well as a preventative treatment. It relieves the blockages in your energy flow and opens the circulation of your life force before physical symptoms appear.

Imagine two batteries. One has been in your transistor radio for a few months. Your radio does not play as well as it should. It picks up static and the volume won't go very high. You know it's time to change the battery. You find a fresh one and get ready to change it. You open your radio and take out the old battery and put it on the table. The batteries are now lying side by side. The phone rings. It's your Aunt Maude wanting to tell you all about her latest operation. You listen patiently, wish her a speedy recovery, and go back to the task at hand. Now, which is the new battery? They look just the same. The only way you can tell which is which is to put one in the radio and see what happens.

Your body works the same way. Your energy "battery" could be running very low, but your body would look fine. Maybe your "volume" is down. "I'm not feeling myself today," is a common comment from a person whose battery is running low. What if you leave the spent battery in your radio? You forget it there for a year or so? You would open your radio and find corrosion or leaking battery juice. Again, the same thing happens in your body. If your battery is left to get weaker and weaker, then eventually you will see the damage in the form of physical symptoms.

The majority of people on this planet know about the existence of chi. For people raised in Western culture, however, chi is a strange notion; a matter of belief rather than knowledge. People in the West are beginning to recognize that acupuncture works, but, because they were raised in the Western system, try to find an explanation through that system to justify their observation that acupuncture and other forms of alternative medicine work. That is like trying to find English words in a Chinese text. You can't. If you explain how it works through the Chinese system, then it makes perfect sense (as do many other natural occurrences that baffle the Western trained mind).

My mother-in-law's dentist told her, "I don't believe in acupuncture." I had to smile when she said this. To me, it's like hearing somebody say, "I don't believe in gravity." Not so long ago the majority of people in our culture knew the world was flat and that the sun and all the planets revolved around the earth. The few people who believed otherwise and had the courage (or audacity) to express their opinions got into *big trouble!*

As technology developed and broadened our vision (the invention of the telescope, for instance), our cultural norms changed. Now, everybody knows that the earth is round. What else have we learned lately about the earth? What about the science of ecology? Ecology was a word that most of our parents never heard when they were growing up. Now every child in school can tell you what it means. There is a cultural awareness about the necessity to preserve the planet by realizing the impact that separate things have on the whole.

Let's consider, for a moment, our "personal ecology." Imagine that your body is the earth. Around the earth is a protective layer called "the atmosphere." Your body has the same thing. It is called an "aura" or "etheric body." Just as pollutants produced on the earth can create a hole in its atmosphere, a weakness in your system (caused by internal factors like stress, emotional upsets, or an improper diet, or external influences such as exposure to strong underground vibrations, or electromagnetic vibration from your television, computers, or cell phones) can cause a hole in your protective shield. The hole itself is not the problem. It's what can come in through the hole that can do the damage. In the case of the earth, it's harmful cosmic rays, ultraviolet rays, or x-rays. In the case of your body, it's viruses and bacteria, which are always around us. Why is it that some people are affected by them and others are not? Ever wondered?

If you would like to experience the chi flow in your body, try this simple exercise:

Sit or stand comfortably. Take a deep breath to calm yourself. With your elbows close to your sides, hold your forearms so they are parallel to the floor. Turn your palms to face one another. Take another deep breath. Keep breathing deeply while you *slowly* bring your palms together. When your palms are about two inches apart, make *slow* circular movements as if you were washing your hands, keeping your palms flat and facing one another. Don't let your hands touch one another; keep them about two inches apart. Feel what's happening. Don't continue reading. Try it!

Did you do it? What did you feel? When your palms were about six to eight inches apart, you probably started to feel a slight pulsing. It's important to keep breathing because breath and chi work together. As you made the circles, did you feel a tingling in your palms? What you felt was chi. That's it.

Think about this: Modern Western medicine has been around for about two hundred years—tops. Chinese medicine has been around for about four thousand years. Modern Western medicine, with its technological aids like microscopes, scanners, machines that breathe for you, and all the other medical wonders, is very good for putting you back together when you are broken. Developments in the fields of molecular biology and immunology have wiped out many previously fatal diseases, saving many lives. However, when it comes to quality of health and preventative medicine, the Western way is off the mark. It denies the very existence of the parts of your body that are crucial to your vitality—your chi and your aura.

Time and time again I hear stories of people going to the doctor complaining that they "don't feel right." The doctor checks them the "modern" way, finds nothing wrong, and either sends them home with a "Tsk, tsk, it's all in your head," or with some medication to calm them so they don't notice that they are not feeling right. Most likely, these patients have recognized a blockage in their chi. If their chi is strengthened at this stage, it's likely that a more serious problem will be avoided and the day-to-day quality of their lives will be greatly improved, as will their energy levels.

When I was studying in China, a doctor told me, "In the West when you go to a doctor, they ask you about your family history. 'Did your parents suffer from any particular disease, for example?' Here in China, often the patients ask me, 'Is your family healthy? Are you in good health?' If I can't keep myself and my family in good health, why should a person put his life in my hands?"

Your good health is in your hands.

9

△△△△△△△△△△△

P.S. I Love You

Remember our friends, the fish? Now that you have an understanding of the basic idea of the sign, I'd like to explain, in a little more detail, what the sign means.

Do you see the one bit of detail on the fishies? Yes, they each have an eye. It is the opposite color of their bodies. This tells us that within Yin there is Yang, and vice versa.

In winter (Yin), we occasionally enjoy a glorious sunny day (Yang). In summer (Yang), there are sometimes showers (Yin). Within each side is constant movement from extreme to moderate and to the other extreme until it can't go any farther and comes back again. So, Yin and Yang are always in movement, creating a dynamic balance. Imagine the sign rotating around in three dimensions. Beautiful, isn't it? It's the dance of life.

An example of this principle in action is the effect that alcohol has in the human body. Alcohol, as you remember, has Yin energy. When we have one drink we feel relaxed and in a good mood. Relaxed is a Yin state. If we continue to drink, our tongues begin to loosen. We want to find someone to talk to. This phase is beginning to get Yang. It's getting more outgoing, as are we. Yet another drink brings us to a very Yang stage. Depending on our personality, this takes the form of good-natured (though possibly out-of-tune) singing, dancing on the tables, outrageous jokes, or even a fight. The morning after all this partying, the Yin really takes effect. We've come full circle. We want to stay in bed, in the dark, with no loud noises.

Another example of the Yin and Yang from nature is the monthly cycle of the phases of the moon. The full moon, of course, is the most Yang time of the cycle. It has been noted in various studies that more violent crimes are committed at this time. The word *lunatic* comes from *luna,* the Latin word for moon. Someone who was crazy was thought to be under the influence of the moon. I explained before how underground water affects the water in our bodies. Knowing how the moon affects the waters of the oceans in the form of tides, it's not difficult to make the connection that our bodies are also affected by the pull of the moon.

A woman's menstrual cycle is about the same length as one full cycle of the moon. Women who live close to nature and are deeply aware of moon phases generally will menstruate during the new moon. Have you ever noticed that when women live together, their menstrual periods often synchronize? This is the most Yin time of the month. In some Native American cultures, the women of the tribe would spend their menstrual days away from their normal duties. They would spend this time together, not engaging in their everyday Yang activities of preparing food and caring for their families. They would walk in nature and collect medicinal herbs or sit quietly together and tap into the Yin, or feminine energy. Afterward, they would share the insights gained at this time with the rest of the tribe. In today's busy world, we have lost this deep connection with the feminine, magnetic energy. Women, remember this information the next time you get annoyed with "the curse"; use this time consciously to tap into your body's deeper wisdom.

Another familiar example is water. As ice, it is in its extreme point of Yin. In its liquid form, it is at the point of equilibrium—its natural state. As steam, it is at its most Yang—expanded and without form.

Consider a seed: Yin, quiet, self-contained. Add energy in the form of nutrients from the earth and heat from the sun, and it begins its journey toward Yang. It grows to maturity, the most extreme Yang moment of its life cycle. Then it begins the process of returning to the earth, eventually changing back to Yin, and losing its form as a plant; its parts are broken up and recycled back into the earth.

The same goes for us. As children, we are growing with Yang energy. We are active and moving all the time. We need more fuel to help our bodies energize and grow. As we reach maturity, we are at the peak of mental and physical activity. As we age, we become more Yin in nature: calmer, contemplative, and, hopefully, wiser, having learned from past experiences. When thinking about which foods are best for you to eat, take your age into consideration.

Once you are familiar with which foods are Yin and which are Yang, start to think about what happens when you cook them. Preparing food is how we bring it closer to balance. Take frozen vegetables, for example: they are in an extreme state of Yin—there is no movement, no bacteria can grow, and no decay takes place. Fire is an extreme Yang state. Something will burn until there is nothing left but ashes—and ashes are Yin. Again, we've come full circle.

When you cook meat, you make it even more Yang. It crosses the extreme point. When it cools down, it is less Yang then before it was cooked. Amazing. Extreme Yin foods are moderated by being warmed up. On a winter's day, to make a meal more Yang, you can use salt, soy sauce, or hot spices. To balance a meal toward the Yin side, add more fresh vegetables, either raw or lightly cooked. If you understand the logic, it's easy to remember what to eat.

If spicy food is Yang, then why is it that many places with a hot (Yang) climate traditionally use lots of spices? Mexican food uses chili and cumin. Indian cuisine incorporates curry, chili, cardamom, and many other spices. Szechwan food can knock your socks off. Don't the spices plus the hot climate tip the balance too much toward the Yang side? A closer look will show that some hot climates are also very humid. Humidity creates dampness in the body, a Yin condition. The Yang energy of the spices counteracts the dampness.

Also, the extreme Yang of hot weather in addition to spices effectively kills microorganisms that breed like wildfire in hot and humid conditions. In these countries, it is also a tradition to have a siesta after meals. A little nap provides the necessary Yin balance.

If you ever get confused, you can't go wrong if you eat everything in *moderation.*

In chapters 6 and 7 I talked about vibrations. This is a *huge* subject. I would like to mention one more thing that you might have experienced yourself. When you meet a person for the first time, do you sometimes feel really comfortable with that person or sometimes take an instant dislike to them? Do you wonder why? It has to do with a difference between your vibrational field and theirs. There is a resonance or disharmony between your two energetic fields. Sometimes you may feel uncomfortable in a certain place, or in a certain position in a room. The reason is the same—a disharmony between you and the vibrational frequency of your environment. Learn to notice these things. The more sensitive you are to the vibrations around you, the more aware you become of the vast amount of information that is available for the taking, but you must know where to look for it.

Now, I'd like to say a word about nutritional supplements. It seems to me that every year there is a new "fashionable" vitamin, mineral, combination supplement, or "wonder drug" of the herbal world. Certain supplements are useful when you have identified an imbalance in your body and are actively involved in a method of treating this imbalance, but *a supplement is not a substitute* for the nutrients found in food. I always tell my patients that supplements are "secondhand health." You don't want to be secondhand healthy, do you? To become dependent on supplements is yet another "quick fix" and will not lead to long-term health and balance. Used often, mineral supplements, which are extremely Yin, will in themselves cause your body to be out of balance.

To change the subject . . . what is pain? Pain is your body's natural way of letting you know that something is wrong. When a child first touches a flame she gets a burn. She very quickly learns not to touch it again. We learn through experience to avoid contact with things that cause us pain. This happens on an emotional level, as well. Often, a person who has been hurt in a relationship will hold back and limit his feeling the next time. Once bitten, twice shy. As we begin to understand ourselves, our bodies, and our emotions, we can start to free ourselves of the limitations caused by the experience of pain. To simply *know* that pain is a warning sign whose function is to protect you, not an enemy to be conquered, is an important key.

As we start to find our balance and make friends with our bodies, new worlds of understanding and happiness will begin to unfold. Welcome to the adventure of a lifetime.

Bon voyage and happy trails!

10

△△△△△△△△△△△

The End of the Beginning

You now have a greater understanding of your bodies, both physical and etheric, and how they interact with your environment.

Your body is your greatest teacher and healer. If you learn to quiet your mind, let go of all the advertising hype, and listen to the wisdom of your body, it's simple to be healthy.

Now you know that your health depends on many things and that, though popping a pill may make you feel better for a while, *true and lasting health depends on you taking responsibility for your body.* That's what this book is about: *your responsibility!*

Where do you start to make the change? You already have, my friends, by reading this book. You now have all the information and tools that you need to take another step on the road to good health.

Think about the food that you put into your body. Consider the weather and your level of activity. Try to eat fresh foods that are in season where you live. You'll know what's in season by the price. Fruit and vegetables that are in season are cheaper. If your current eating habits are a long way from ideal, slowly start to make changes. It may take some time to change the foods that you've been eating and enjoying for years, so don't feel you have to do it all at once. Start by avoiding extreme foods and eating more of the things that are closer to the center of the seesaw—take another look at the food chart on the following page. It's okay to *occasionally* eat something you really enjoy but that you know is not particularly good for you, but don't keep unhealthy food in your home—simply don't buy it! Let's say you feel a craving for a donut; ask yourself, "Do I really want this *now?*" (The key word here is *now.*) If you can wait, then don't eat it. There are plenty of donuts in the world. If you *really* want one, then you can go and get one. Get out of the habit of eating things just because they are there without asking your body if it really wants it. It's that simple.

Avoid processed foods. In affluent countries, people often have more money than time. A whole industry exists to provide "convenience" food to save the cook time and effort, but pay attention to the ingredients listed on the package of this food. The list of ingredients often reads more like a chemistry book than a cookbook. Some companies are now beginning to make products with fewer preservatives, but the only way to really know what you are eating is to make it yourself. Buy the freshest and least processed foods you can. Organic foods produced without the use of pesticides or hormones are the best. They may seem more expensive, but in the long run they are cost effective. You get better quality food—more nutrients for the same quantity of food. You will eat less because your body will get the nutrition it needs. In addition, you'll find that your shopping bills actually go down and, if you are on the heavy side, your weight will probably go down, too.

If you wake up feeling tired every morning, move your bed. Ask a friend to help you use the muscle test (see appendix B) to find a better spot for it. Leave it in the new place for ten days to two weeks. If you are still waking up feeling tired, move your bed again. If you cannot move it, then get some stones as mentioned in chapter 7 and put them under your mattress in order to protect yourself against the negative vibrations. Once you find a place where you can sleep well, *make sure you sleep enough.* Give your body a chance to renew and rebuild itself during your hours of sleep.

Be aware of electromagnetic fields in your environment. Move all electrical equipment away from your bed. Check the other side of the wall near the head of your bed. If there is a fuse box, circuit breaker, computer, or microwave oven there, *move your bed.* When working on a computer, take frequent breaks for fresh air. Look into devices that neutralize the effects of harmful environmental vibrations.

Learn to relax and take it easy. Watch your body when strong emotions threaten to push you off balance. *Remember to breathe.*

Get more oxygen into your blood by walking in nature; walk in unspoiled rural areas if you can, or in a park. Listen to the birds. Find a sport, dance class, or any physical activity that you enjoy and participate on a regular basis.

Drink pure spring water. Sometimes tap water contains chemicals that can be harmful to your system. It's better to drink pure spring water whenever you can. It's inexpensive and often tastes much better!

Find things you like to do and do them. If you are in a job that you hate, think about changing jobs or find an aspect of it that you enjoy and try to get in a position where you will spend more of your time doing that. If you can't change jobs, then make time for a hobby that really gives you pleasure. If you can't think of anything you like to do, think back to what you enjoyed as a child: model-making, playing with trains or dolls, climbing trees. You can still make models, collect trains, or start a doll hospital to repair a child's treasure. If tree-climbing is your thing, remember that you may be a little heavier now than you were a decade or two ago, so choose a tree with strong branches. You know you've found something you love doing when hours pass without you realizing it.

Turn off the television. Or better still, don't turn it on. If the first thing that you do when you get up in the morning is turn on the television, get out of that habit. Find a radio station that plays music you like. Avoid news-only and talk stations and listen to music stations—you'll still get enough news and traffic to find out what you need to know. Better yet, listen to a tape, a CD, or enjoy silence. When you listen to the news and advertisements, be discerning. Don't believe everything you hear, and don't let the information avalanche throw you off balance.

Spend time with people you like. And I don't mean sitting around a television set. Get to know other people. Go out and play together. Go for walks or join in sporting or social events. Spend your time with positive people and the kind of people you would like to be yourself. If your current situation means that you have to spend time with people whose company you don't enjoy, you may have to make some changes. As you get healthier, you might find that people who you thought were friends resent the fact that you are developing yourself. You may seem too independent and they may feel that you no longer need them for support now that you are taking responsibility for yourself. These people are not *real* friends. A real friend wishes the best for you. As you become healthier, you will meet others who are walking the same road—a road that, down the line, leads to a much happier life. You will see that the journey itself is the exciting part—the things you learn, the people you meet, the fun you have on the way—not just the eventual destination.

Life is a dynamic exchange of Yin and Yang. Sometimes we have good days, sometimes bad days, and some days are right in the middle. Bad days are our teachers. They give us an opportunity to see what is not working in our lives. Once we are aware of what that is, we can do something to change it. As you make the necessary changes, you will find that the bad days will become fewer and the bad things that happen are not really *so* bad. Be patient.

When we have a good day, we can share our happiness and energy with others. A kind act or even the sight of a smiling face can start a pleasant chain reaction in the world that can have consequences beyond imagination.

Fill your emotional quota with happiness and share it with others. The more you give, the more you will get back.

Appendix A

▲▲▲▲▲▲▲▲▲▲▲

In the Kitchen

I have suggested that one way of balance is through your stomach. Besides understanding the principles of Yin and Yang, I want you to also consider the act of preparing and eating your food. If you cook or eat in a rush, you lose many of the benefits of your food. Why? In a word, *stress.* Our busy, contemporary lifestyles create stress and worry that affect the stomach, whose job is to separate "impure" energy from "pure" energy; that is, the nutrients from the waste products. If you want to get the most from your food, take your time preparing and eating it; connect yourself with your "fuel."

Before you prepare a meal, set your cooking "stage." Make your kitchen a pleasant place to be. Keep it clean, tidy, and free of clutter. Have some flowers or herbs growing by the window. Put on some music that you enjoy. When you cut your vegetables, think about how they grew from a tiny seed into something delicious and nourishing. If you cook meat, thank the animal for providing you with nourishment. Balance your body, mind, and spirit as you cook. Infuse your ingredients with happiness—singing in the kitchen makes everything taste better. Don't take my word for it. Try it and see.

As I mentioned before, when you eat, don't watch television or read the newspaper. Focus on the food you eat and on the good company you are sharing it with.

Here are four simple and delicious recipes that not only please the palate, but the nose and eyes as well.

Donna Mariana's Magic Soup

In Yugoslavia, we always have soup as our first course with lunch. Here is the basic recipe.

½ large onion, minced
1 large carrot, grated
1 stock cube
½ cup uncooked rice
1 tablespoon vegetable oil
5 cups filtered water
½ cup peas, chopped mushrooms,
    or celery (in addition to or
    instead of the rice), optional

Sauté the onions in the oil over medium-high heat. When they dry out and become translucent, add the carrots and cook for a few more minutes.

Add the water and the stock cube (crumbled). Bring to a boil. Add rice and vegetables and simmer until they become soft, about 10 to 15 minutes.

Season with freshly ground black pepper, a little dill, or chopped parsley. To make the soup a little more Yang, add soy sauce. To make it a little more Yin, add a small amount of vinegar.

This soup is particularly good for you at the time of year when the seasons change. It supports your stomach and spleen and keeps your digestive system in good condition.

Serves 4

The Famous 3-2-1 Combo

This combination is familiar to all my patients. It is a wonderful blood tonic and a superb energizer. If you don't feel well, have a little every day, otherwise once a week is enough. There are two ways to enjoy the benefits of this combination. One is as a salad and the other is as juice. Why 3-2-1? Because you will need:

> 3 red things: beets, apples, carrots
> 2 green things: celery, parsley
> 1 yellow thing: a lemon

For juice: Put one beet, one apple, one or two carrots, a stalk of celery, a little parsley, and half a lemon through your juicer. You can vary the amounts to taste. Sip a glassful after meals.

For a salad: Grate the beet, apple, and carrots. Chop the celery and the parsley. Use the juice of the lemon to make a dressing with a little olive oil. Garnish with walnuts. The oil helps your body to absorb the vitamins and minerals. Try this at home. It tastes much better than it sounds!

The Chinese say, "Satisfy your eyes with colors." Translation: If you eat a variety of foods, something of every color, then your nutritional needs will be met.

If you use one of each item, you will get 2 large glasses of juice or enough salad for 4 servings; feel free to use more of what you like best

Warning: The first time you drink this juice or eat this salad, your body will probably absorb all the nutrients in the beets. However, the second or third time, your body won't need so much and the result will be bright pink liquid waste! Don't panic if you see what looks like blood in the toilet; it's just the excess beet juice being eliminated.

Note from Francesca: I always hated beets. When Igor suggested that I eat them to strengthen my system, at first I thought, "No way!" But slowly, slowly, I began to eat cooked beets when I saw them at salad bars. (The first time I ate them I had a cold and couldn't taste anything.) Eventually, they didn't seem so bad. When I tried them raw, grated in this salad, I really liked them. Now I eat them often with real enjoyment—and I feel a lot better, too.

Old Fashioned Gingersnaps

When the winter winds blow and the sky is gray and drizzly, the ginger and cinnamon in these delicious cookies will warm you right down to your toes. Make a double batch of dough and keep some in the refrigerator (before you roll it out)—pop a few cookies at a time in the oven and fill your kitchen with the soothing smell of homemade goodies.

2¼ cups flour
½ teaspoon cinnamon
1 teaspoon ginger
⅓ cup butter
½ cup brown sugar
1 egg, well beaten
½ cup molasses
2 teaspoons baking soda

Preheat the oven to 350 degrees.

Mix the flour, cinnamon, and ginger together.

Cream butter and gradually add the sugar, beating until light. Add beaten egg and molasses.

Dissolve baking soda in 2 teaspoons of hot water and add to the creamed mixture.

Combine the dry ingredients and creamed mixture. Chill.

Roll out on a lightly floured board to ⅛-inch thickness and cut into fun shapes with cookie cutters. Place cookies on a greased baking sheet.

Bake for 10 to 12 minutes.

Makes about 3 dozen medium-sized cookies

Francesca's "Secret" Hot Mulled Wine

Good for the holidays and cold weather. It will promote circulation and warm up your body. To soothe away PMS (premenstrual syndrome), drink one cupful every evening when the first symptoms appear. Keep the rest in the refrigerator for up to a week. Heat it up and drink as needed.

> 1 cup water
> ¾ cup brown sugar
> 4–5 cinnamon sticks
> 1–2 lemons, sliced thin
> 30 cloves, whole
> 1 bottle red wine

Stick the whole cloves firmly into the lemon slices.

Combine sugar, water, and cinnamon in a saucepan. Place over a low heat. Just after it reaches the boiling point, lower the heat and simmer for 5 minutes.

Pour the mixture over the lemon slices studded with cloves and let stand at least 30 minutes.

Add the wine. Heat very slowly to just under the boiling point. Add a little boiling water to dilute the wine, if you like.

Strain and serve nice and hot. Cheers!

Serves 6 to 8

Appendix B

World Famous
Muscle Test

To do this "test," you will need either a suitcase that is *almost* too heavy for you to lift, or a friend. This test is based on the premise "your body never lies."

Your body can show you which places are affected by harmful waves. You'll be able to detect places affected by underground waves or electromagnetic fields.

Have your friend stand facing you; extend her right arm straight from the shoulder, parallel with the floor. Press down *slowly and evenly* on her forearm, while she resists you with all her strength. This is not a contest to see who is stronger, so take it easy! Both you and your friend should be able to feel the point where it's difficult to resist the pressure.

Maybe you won't be able to push her arm down at all! I have a friend who is a professional body builder. I tried the test on him, in a place that was not affected by harmful waves. I could practically do chin-ups on his outstretched arm. Then we went to quiet corner of his gym, an area where nobody liked to work out. I had checked the space before and knew that it was influenced by an underground stream. We tried the test there. You should have seen his face when I pressed his arm down with two fingers. It's sad to see a grown man cry!

If you can easily push your friend's arm down, move to another spot; the first one might not be "clear." If you are much stronger, ask your friend to push your arm while you resist. Once you've established the amount of resistance in a clear spot, it's time to try it in an area where there are harmful waves. Have you friend stand with her back to a television set. Try the test with the set turned on and with it turned off. See what happens.

Test the places where you spend a lot of time: your desk, your television chair, and the most important place of all, your bed. Move the bed out of the way and do the muscle test where your head would be, and then all the way down to your feet. If your resistance is low, *move your bed!* Find a spot where your arm stays strong.

If you can't find a friend to help you with this, do it by yourself. Fill a suitcase until you can just about hold it in one hand when your arm is extended out to one side of your body at shoulder height. Move around to different locations; if you can hold it without discomfort, then the place is good. If it is too heavy to lift, then the place is not good. Don't do this test too many times in a row; your arm may get sore.

You can do this test with other things, too. Test a cell phone, tobacco, or chocolate, and watch what happens. Try a banana or a tomato. Hold the item in question in your left hand, over your heart. Have your friend press on your arm, as before. You can test different foods, drugs, or vitamins to see which ones can help you and which may harm you. Try the same thing on different days. What's bad for you on Monday might be okay on Thursday. Some things are always a no-no. Find out which ones and avoid them. Try this at your next party. The stronger the "victim" the better. Cell phones are always good for a laugh.

△△△△△△△△△△△

Suggested Reading List

To learn more about how your body works:
Parker, Steve. *The Body Atlas, A Pictorial Guide to the Human Body.* London, Great Britain: Dorling Kindersley, 1993.

A lighthearted but thorough explanation of Yin & Yang:
Go. *The Tao of Baseball.* Fireside, 1991.

A wonderful book that can help you get in touch with the cycles of nature and your own hidden wisdom:
Parry, Danaan. *The Essene Book of Days.* Seattle, Washington: Earth Stewards Network, 1997.

How your emotions influence your health:
Hay, Louise. *You Can Heal Your Life.* Hay House, 1984.

A good book about diet:

Jingfeng, Cai. *Eating Your Way to Health, Dietotherapy in Traditional Chinese Medicine.* Beijing, China: Foreign Language Press, 1988.

A very good resource for educational information on all sorts of conditions:

Rector Page, Linda, N.D., Ph.D. *Healthy Healing, A Guide to Self Healing for Everyone.* Healthy Healing Publications, 1997.

To learn more about your chakras:

Brennan, Barbara Ann. *Hands of Light, A Guide to Healing Through the Human Energy Field.* New York, New York: Bantam Books, 1987.

Some good books about the healing properties of crystals and gemstones:

Harold, Edmund. *Focus on Crystals.* New York, New York: Ballantine Books, 1987.

Gem Elixirs and Vibrational Healing. Vol. II, Gurudas, Cassandra Press, 1989.

Chocron, Daya Sarai. *Healing with Crystals and Gemstones.* York Beach, Maine: Samuel Weiser, Inc. 1988.

Everything you ever wanted to know about vibrational medicine:

Gerber, Richard, M.D. *Vibrational Medicine, New Choices of Healing Ourselves.* Santa Fe, New Mexico: Bear & Company, 1988.

Bibliography

Beinfield, Harriet, L.Ac. and Efram Korngold, L.Ac., O.M.D. *Between Heaven And Earth, A Guide to Chinese Medicine.* New York, New York: Ballantine Books, 1992.

Becker, Robert O., M.D. *Cross Currents, The Promise of Electromedicine.* New York, New York: Penguin Putnam, Inc., 1990.

Becker, Robert O., M.D., and Gary Selden. *The Body Electric: Electromagnetism and The Foundation of Life.* New York, New York: Quill, William Morrow, 1985.

Kuan, Dr. Hin. *Chinese Massage and Acupressure.* New York, New York: Berg Publishing, Inc., 1991.

Lu, Henry C. *Chinese Foods For Longevity, The Art of Long Life.* New York, New York: Sterling Publishing Company, Inc., 1990.

Michio, Kushi. *Your Face Never Lies.* New Jersey: Avery Publishing Group, 1983.

Thurnel-Read, Jane. *Geopathic Stress: How Earth Energies Affect Our Lives.* London, Great Britain: Element Books Ltd., 1995.

REACH FOR THE MOON

Llewellyn publishes hundreds of books on your favorite subjects! To get these exciting books, including the ones on the following pages, check your local bookstore or order them directly from Llewellyn.

ORDER BY PHONE

- Call toll-free within the U.S. and Canada, 1-800-THE MOON
- In Minnesota, call (651) 291-1970
- We accept VISA, MasterCard, and American Express

ORDER BY MAIL

- Send the full price of your order (MN residents add 7% sales tax) in U.S. funds, plus postage & handling to:

  Llewellyn Worldwide
  P.O. Box 64383, Dept. K1-56718-121-X
  St. Paul, MN 55164–0383, U.S.A.

POSTAGE & HANDLING
(For the U.S., Canada, and Mexico)

- $4.00 for orders $15.00 and under
- $5.00 for orders over $15.00
- No charge for orders over $100.00

We ship UPS in the continental United States. We ship standard mail to P.O. boxes. Orders shipped to Alaska, Hawaii, The Virgin Islands, and Puerto Rico are sent first-class mail. Orders shipped to Canada and Mexico are sent surface mail.

International orders: Airmail—add freight equal to price of each book to the total price of order, plus $5.00 for each non-book item (audio tapes, etc.).

Surface mail—Add $1.00 per item.

Allow 2 weeks for delivery on all orders.
Postage and handling rates subject to change.

DISCOUNTS

We offer a 20% discount to group leaders or agents. You must order a minimum of 5 copies of the same book to get our special quantity price.

FREE CATALOG

Get a free copy of our color catalog, New Worlds of Mind and Spirit. Subscribe for just $10.00 in the United States and Canada ($30.00 overseas, airmail). Many bookstores carry New Worlds—ask for it!

Visit our website at www.llewellyn.com for more information.

The Art of Spiritual Healing
Chakra and Energy Bodywork

KEITH SHERWOOD

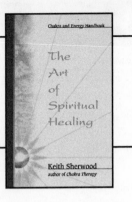

Each of you has the potential to be a healer; to heal yourself and to become a channel for healing others. Healing energy is always flowing through you. Learn how to recognize and tap this incredible energy source. You do not need to be a victim of disease or poor health. Rid yourself of negativity and become a channel for positive healing.

Become acquainted with your three auras and learn how to recognize problems and heal them on a higher level before they become manifested in the physical body as disease.

Special techniques make this book a "breakthrough" to healing power, but you are also given a concise, easy-to-follow regimen of good health to follow in order to maintain a superior state of being. This is a practical guide to healing.

0-87542-720-0
224 pp., 5¼ x 8, illus.   **$9.95**

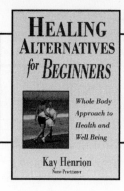

Healing Alternatives for Beginners
*Whole Body Approach to Health
and Well-Being*

KAY HENRION

When someone begins to seek out alternative ways of healing, they encounter a deluge of confusing and often conflicting information on health, healing modalities, foods, and supplements, even from the practitioners themselves.

This book, written by a registered nurse, gives people a starting place for their journey into taking responsibility for their own health. It answers questions in layman's language regarding meditation and visualization, diets and vitamins, herbs, homeopathy, therapeutic touch, the aging process, AIDS, and there's even a chapter about natural healing for pets. It is full of anecdotes and examples from the author's own life and the lives of her patients.

1-56718-427-8
264 pp., 5³⁄₁₆ x 8 $12.95

Chinese Health Care Secrets
A Natural Lifestyle Approach

Henry Lin

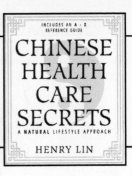

At a time when the medical costs in this country are skyrocket-
ing and chronic disease runs rampant in every walk of life, Chinese Health Care Secrets offers a readily applicable, completely
natural, and highly effective alternative. It serves as a practical
reference on personal health care, as well as a textbook on a
health care system from the world's oldest civilization.

It is the Chinese belief that you can achieve optimal health
by carrying out your daily activities—including diet, sleep,
emotional feeling, physical exercise, and sexual activity—
according to the laws of Nature. It is especially effective in
treating the degenerative diseases that plague millions of
Americans.

Many of the techniques have never before been published,
and are considered secrets even in China.

1-56718-434-0
528 pp., 7½ x 9⅛, illus. $24.95

To order, call 1-800-THE MOON
Prices subject to change without notice

Chi Gung
Chinese Healing, Energy and Natural Magick

L. V. Carnie

Chi Gung is unlike any other magickal book that you've read. There are no spells, incantations, or special outfits. Instead, you will learn more than eighty different exercises that will help you to tap into the magickal power of universal energy. This power, called Chi in Chinese, permeates everything in existence; you can direct the flow of Chi to help you achieve ultimate health as well as any of your dreams and desires.

Chi Gung uses breathing, postures, and increased sensory awareness exercises that follow a particular training program. Ultimately, you can manipulate Chi without focusing on your breathing or moving your muscles in specific patterns. In fact, eventually you can learn how to move and transmit Chi instantly, anywhere, anytime, using only your mind.

1-56718-113-9
256 pp., 7 x 10, illus. $17.50

The Healer's Manual
*A Beginners Guide to
Energy Therapies*

TED ANDREWS

Did you know that a certain Mozart symphony can ease digestion problems . . . that swelling often indicates being stuck in
outworn patterns . . . that breathing pink is good for skin conditions and loneliness? Most dis-ease stems from a metaphys-
ical base. While we are constantly being exposed to viruses
and bacteria, it is our unbalanced or blocked emotions, atti-
tudes, and thoughts that deplete our natural physical energies
and make us more susceptible to "catching a cold" or mani-
festing some other physical problem.

Healing, as approached in The Healer's Manual, involves
locating and removing energy blockages wherever they
occur—physical or otherwise. This book is an easy guide to
simple vibrational healing therapies that anyone can learn to
apply to restore homeostasis to their body's energy system. By
employing sound, color, fragrance, etheric touch, and
flower/gem elixers, you can participate actively within the
healing of your body and the opening of higher perceptions.
You will discover that you can heal more aspects of your life
than you ever thought possible.

0-87542-007-9
256 pp., 6 x 9, illus. $12.95

To order, call 1-800-THE MOON
Prices subject to change without notice